**FOR**

# HEALTHCARE
# RESEARCH

Volume I: Basic Statistical Methods

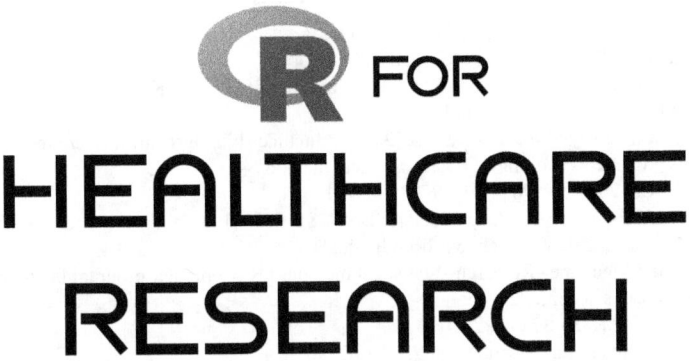

# HEALTHCARE RESEARCH

## Volume I: Basic Statistical Methods

**Jason L. Oke**
*University of Oxford, UK*

**Mei-Man Lee**
*University of Bath, UK*

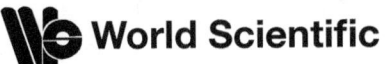 **World Scientific**

NEW JERSEY · LONDON · SINGAPORE · BEIJING · SHANGHAI · HONG KONG · TAIPEI · CHENNAI · TOKYO

*Published by*

World Scientific Publishing Europe Ltd.

57 Shelton Street, Covent Garden, London WC2H 9HE

*Head office:* 5 Toh Tuck Link, Singapore 596224

*USA office:* 27 Warren Street, Suite 401-402, Hackensack, NJ 07601

**Library of Congress Cataloging-in-Publication Data**

Names: Oke, Jason L. author | Lee, Mei-Man author
Title: R for healthcare research / Jason L. Oke, University of Oxford, UK,
   Mei-Man Lee, University of Bath, UK.
Description: New Jersey : World Scientific, [2026]- | Includes bibliographical references
   and index. | Contents: Volume I. Basic statistical methods --
Identifiers: LCCN 2025009596 | ISBN 9781800617186 vol. 1 hardcover |
   ISBN 9781800617315 vol. 1 paperback | ISBN 9781800617193 vol. 1 ebook for institutions |
   ISBN 9781800617209 vol. 1 ebook for individuals
Subjects: LCSH: Medicine--Research--Statistical methods | R (Computer program language) |
   Medical statistics--Computer programs
Classification: LCC R853.S7 O44 2026
LC record available at https://lccn.loc.gov/2025009596

**British Library Cataloguing-in-Publication Data**
A catalogue record for this book is available from the British Library.

R logo © 2016 The R Foundation, distributed under a CC BY-SA 4.0 license
(https://creativecommons.org/licenses/by-sa/4.0/)

For any available supplementary material, please visit
https://www.worldscientific.com/worldscibooks/10.1142/Q0506#t=suppl

Desk Editors: Nambirajan Karuppiah/Gabriel Rawlinson/Shi Ying Koe

Typeset by Stallion Press
Email: enquiries@stallionpress.com

# Foreword

There are many ways of thinking about statistics: as a branch of applied mathematics, as the natural 'scientific language', or, less charitably, as a means of justifying any conclusion one wishes to promote – the often-quoted 'lies, damned lies, and statistics', a phrase popularised by Mark Twain. My own view is that this last characterisation arises from a lack of understanding and appreciation of both the strengths and the limitations of the discipline.

This book provides a carefully designed pathway for understanding and conducting statistical analyses using R, with a particular focus on clinical research. The recent advent of large language models (LLMs), such as ChatGPT, has made access to coding and to the rudiments of analysis and interpretation available to a far wider audience. Yet, the central challenge remains: one must still ask the right questions and, critically, evaluate whether the answers are correct – or at least plausible. This book offers a superb entry point, equipping readers to appreciate the possibilities of statistical analysis, to recognise its constraints, and to navigate its fundamental options.

The primary audience is graduate students with a basic grounding in statistical methods for medical research, but the scope is broader. Clinical practitioners, early-career researchers, and statisticians seeking to engage more directly with clinical applications will all find this book of considerable value. Its emphasis is on application, but it contains just the right amount of theory to remind us why assumptions matter, how to assess whether they are met, and which assumptions are most critical. For instance, the discussion of hypothesis testing versus hypothesis-generating analysis, together with the caution against overloading a study with pre-specified hypotheses (and thereby eroding statistical power), is especially instructive.

Each chapter is structured around clear objectives and learning outcomes. Through a well-balanced combination of text, figures, and R code, the reader is guided from the rationale for a particular analysis to its practical implementation, to the presentation of results, and finally to their interpretation. The worked examples are grounded in real data, drawn from nearly two decades of applied research. At its heart lies a principle shared by most statisticians: *that we must always consider how the data were collected or sampled and to whom the findings can legitimately be generalised.*

Dr Jason Oke brings to this book nearly two decades of experience as a practising medical statistician and researcher, along with more than a decade of teaching undergraduate and graduate students. It reflects the gap he has repeatedly observed: the need for a clear, practice-oriented guide to statistical analyses in R for those working with clinical data.

One of the book's major strengths is its clarity of exposition and its accessible style, which encourage readers to begin analysing data both quickly and accurately. The treatment of $p$-values – clarifying their appropriate interpretation and highlighting common misuses – is a case in point. The book assumes some prior familiarity with statistical concepts, but its design, with examples and end-of-chapter problems, allows readers both to consolidate their learning and to test their understanding. These exercises will challenge even those who already consider themselves well-versed in the subject.

In short, this book represents the distillation of years of thought and practice into a resource that sits elegantly between a theoretical text on statistical methods and a clinically oriented manual. Chapters such as the one on clinical measurement and the discussion distinguishing between statistical significance and clinical importance illustrate this bridging function perfectly. Whether read systematically from cover to cover or consulted selectively as a reference, it is an invaluable companion for those seeking to perform sound analyses and to check that their assumptions hold.

On a personal note, I am delighted to see this work come to fruition. It is the product of long effort and dedication, and it achieves its aim with remarkable clarity and good humour. My hope is that this volume will be followed by a sequel, one that carries the same accessible style into the realm of more advanced methods.

*Rafael Perera*
3 September 2025

# Preface

The last 100 years have seen considerable advances in our under-standing of human health and medicine. The true causes of several important diseases, such as cervical cancer, have been identified, and some long-held but incorrect causes of diseases have been overturned. We now know that it is not stress or diet that causes most cases of gastritis and peptic ulcer disease but the bacterium *Helicobacter pylori*. New and effective treatments have been developed, revolution-ising the care for many conditions, and unsafe or ineffective therapies have been withdrawn. More recently, technological advances have led to dramatic changes in how diseases are detected and diagnosed, in some cases, long before symptoms appear.

Statistics have played an integral role in many of these develop-ments by providing a framework that enables clear and precise com-munication of objective scientific evidence – 'a grammar of science', if you will. But we should not be complacent; there remain many important diseases for which the cause is unknown or uncertain. The search for safer, more effective therapies is ongoing, and significant challenges remain in using new diagnostic technology. To solve these problems, researchers should use statistics and statistical thinking in every stage of health research, from planning experiments and trials to disseminating research to the broader public. We hope that this book helps researchers use statistics effectively.

   R is an environment for statistical computing.[1] It is not strictly
a statistical software package like Stata or SPSS. You may need to
do more work to obtain a similar result from a dedicated statistical
software package such as SPSS or Stata. This, in turn, can require
a greater appreciation of what is being calculated, which we think is
not a bad thing, as this often leads to greater understanding!

   So, why should health researchers choose R? While many excellent
commercial stats packages are available, they are often prohibitively
expensive and can be slow to adopt the latest methods and techniques. In contrast, R is free and open source. Although developed
by a core group of expert statisticians, its strength lies in the contri-
butions of researchers and scientists from many different disciplines
and backgrounds from around the world.

*J. L. Oke*

---

[1]The R project began as an alternative to the S language by Ross Ihaka and
Robert Gentleman at the University of Auckland, New Zealand. The first official
'stable beta' version (v1.0) was released on 29 February 2000.

# Acknowledgements

This book would not have been possible without the help of many people. First, I would like to thank our publisher, Laurent Chaminade, and our editors, Rosie Williamson and Gabriel Rawlinson at World Scientific Publishing. Without Laurent's enduring patience and guidance – given over coffee while in the maths department canteen at Oxford – this project may have never got off the ground. We thank Gabriel for expertly seeing this project through to the end. We are also very grateful to the colleagues and clinical investigators we have worked with over the years, from whom we have learnt and whose work we have drawn upon for the examples in this book. These include, but are not limited to, Rafael Perera, Richard Stevens, Thomas Fanshawe, Jenny Hirst, Constantinos Koshiaris, Brian Nicholson, Phil Turner, Benjamin Feakins, Kiana Collins, Alex Novak, Sarim Ather, Jeremy Howick, Carl Heneghan, Roger Kim, and Nicholas Jones.

Jason thanks his wife, Caroline, and his two children, Charlie and Ellie for being the inspiration to carry on working on the book when it all seemed impossible.

M.-M. Lee would like to thank her husband for support and encourage while writing this book.

# About the authors

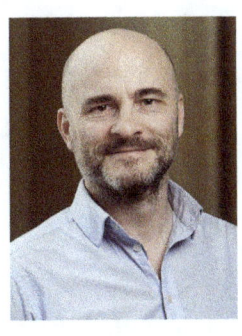

**Jason L. Oke** is a department lecturer in medical statistics and cancer research at the Nuffield Department of Primary Care Health Sciences and a senior associate tutor at the Department of Continuing Education at the University of Oxford. He lectures and teaches evidence-based healthcare and medical statistics with R to undergraduate and postgraduate students. He has co-authored over 150 peer-reviewed research articles with a focus on diagnostics, monitoring, and screening for disease. He is the director of Oxford Biostatistics, an academic contract research organisation specialising in supporting academic research groups and biotechnology companies who develop and assess novel diagnostic technology.

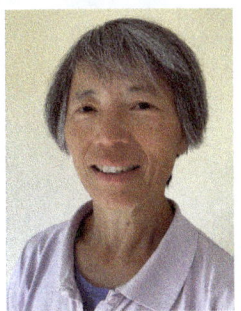

**Mei-Man Lee** is a teaching assistant at the University of Bath. She was formerly a medical statistician at the University of Oxford, with particular expertise in the applications of statistical modelling in healthcare research. She taught statistics and R programming to undergraduate and postgraduate students.

# Contents

# List of figures

# List of tables

## Chapter 1

# Introduction to the R software

R is language and an environment for statistical computing, data manipulation and graphics. It is free and open-source and runs on all standard computing platforms and operating systems. R is based on a simple and effective programming language, and contains an integrated collection of tools and functions for data handling, analysis and creating graphs. In this chapter, we provide a concise introduction to the R language and the key functions required for healthcare research.

**Objectives and learning outcomes**

The objectives for this chapter are to:

- introduce the R computing environment and its basic features
- describe the building blocks of the R language
- outline some practical aspects of elementary programming in R
- show how R can be extended using user-contributed packages

After reading this chapter, you should be able to:

- use R interactively to enter data, and prepare it for analysis
- recognise the different data types and objects used in R
- write scripts/programs and save them as files
- load and use, built-in and external packages/data

## 1.1   R: An environment for statistical programming

R is an environment for statistical computing or programming. The R
system comprises a base R system containing all of the fundamental
functions required for statistics, data manipulation, and graphics. If
this wasn't enough, the base system can be extended by adding one
or more of the thousands of packages contributed by many different
authors. In fact, a great appeal of R is the community of users who
contribute packages and provide solutions to vexing coding problems.
A potential trade-off is that there is 'absolutely no warranty' – a
warning that greets you each time you open R:

```
R is free software and comes with ABSOLUTELY NO WARRANTY.
You are welcome to redistribute it under certain conditions.
Type 'license()' or 'licence()' for distribution details.
```

How worried should we be about this? In our experience, we do
not find this to be a problem. The core functions in base R have
been used for many years and have stood the test of time. Because
of this, R can hold its own among the very best commercial software
and often surpasses the competition. For example, Gallagher (2006)
compared the $p$-values from a two-sided $F$ test across eight different
statistical software packages. Five of the tested packages, including
SAS and Stata, returned the wrong $p$-values, whereas R, along with
S-Plus and Minitab, returned the correct $p$-values.

The R interface is simple, with only a few drop-down menus.
Unlike other statistical packages, you will not find the names of famil-
iar statistical routines among them. This means you will need to
learn the language of R and learn to write out a set of instructions
for R to interpret. While we recognise that this can be intimidat-
ing to start with, we believe the investment in the early stages will
pay dividends in the long run. We start at the beginning, assuming no prior knowledge of computing or programming. By the end
of the book, you will be able to carry out some of the most important statistical techniques required for healthcare research using the
R software.

### 1.1.1 *Scope of the book*

There are many excellent textbooks on the theory of medical statistics and a large number of books and resources dedicated to the R software, but while theoretical books can explain why, they don't show you how analyses can be done in practice. Similarly, whilst there many books on programming R, they tend to omit 'the why' and do not offer much on how to interpret the results. Our aim in this book was combine the 'why' and the 'how' and provide help with the interpretation of the results. The intended audience is the healthcare researcher or student of healthcare research, not necessarily a statistics student. Yet, any student of statistics will appreciate seeing how the methods they have learnt apply in the healthcare setting.

In this book, we cover what we consider to be the most widely used techniques in healthcare research and evidence-based medicine and demonstrate how to carry these out using the R software. Topics covered include displaying data, comparing two samples, determining correlations, and assessing agreement. In addition, we have included explanations of the key ideas and concepts underpinning the analyses used throughout the book, described what data is typically required, the assumptions made, and how these can be checked. Throughout the book, we provide examples from our research and many other research papers we have read while writing this book.

### 1.1.2 *Our preferred method for working with R*

The following points summarise our approach to using R for healthcare research:

- Our work should be reproducible, meaning we will write scripts[1] that document all the steps taken to produce the results.
- We aim to work directly on the source data while always documenting (in a script) any alterations made to them. We avoid making undocumented changes to source data where possible.

---

[1]Files containing our code.

- Our syntax or code will be simple and intuitive, rather than 'elegant' – elegant often means difficult to understand.
- We prefer transparency and interpretability over complexity in general.
- Above all, we aim to get the code right first, and then optimise it, but only if we need to.
- Where we can, we defer to functions from base R to do data manipulation and standard calculations. Although there are many excellent extensions to R, these can change over time, which may prevent your old code from working.
- We prefer to use established statistical methods rather than novel 'sophisticated' approaches.

### 1.1.3   *R examples in this book*

Throughout the book, we provide R code for the examples in shaded boxes, as shown in the following:

```
# Some comment for the R code (not executed)
xy <- x * y
```

Sometimes, we might assume that the R code that appears earlier in the same section of the book has been executed (or run); therefore, to avoid getting frustrating errors, it is advisable to work through the code in the order given in each section.

### 1.1.4   *The R4HCR package*

We have created an R package (R4HCR) containing many of the datasets we refer to in this book. A full explanation of how R packages work and how they are used is given in Section 1.2.4. The R4HCR package is freely available to anyone with an internet connection and can be installed into your library by doing the following:

```
install.packages("R4HCR")

## Installing package into
'/home/user/R/x86_64-pc-linux-gnu-library/4.4'
## (as 'lib' is unspecified)
```

Once installed, you will be able to access the data referred to in the book and recreate the examples and output.

### 1.1.5 *Downloading and installing R*

R can be downloaded from the comprehensive archive network (CRAN) website (https://cran.r-project.org/). Click on one of the links in the *Download and Install R* box. For example, for Windows systems, do the following:

(1) Click on the `Download R for Windows` link.
(2) Click on the `Install R for the first time`.[2]
(3) Finally, click `Download R X.X.X`[3] `for Windows` (62 megabytes, 32/64 bit).

A pop-up box will then appear, stating that you have chosen to open `R-X.X.X-win.exe`, and it asks whether you would like to save this file; click `Save File`. Once downloaded, the `.exe` file can be run by double-clicking on the file name. Follow the instructions for a standard installation.

For Mac, click on the `Download R for macOS` link, and then choose the package (`.pkg`) that matches the Mac OS you are running. Then, click on the `Save file` link. Once downloaded, use Finder to locate the downloaded package, then run it, and follow the instructions. For Linux operating systems, the process is a little more involved and can vary depending on which Linux system you are running, but there is a lot of support on the internet to help with this (e.g., https://linuxtldr.com/installing-r-and-rstudio/).

### 1.1.6 *Integrated development environments*

Although R can be used on its own, you might find it easier to use it with an additional piece of software that is designed to help you organise your workflow. These are grandly titled 'integrated

---

[2]Even if this isn't your first time.
[3]X.X.X = 4.3.1 currently.

development environments', or *IDEs*. They can add functionality, allowing for example, auto-completion of directory paths and functions and other shortcuts. There are many examples, most of which are free, such as RKward (https://rkward.kde. org/), Tinn-R (https://sourceforge.net/projects/tinn-r/, and RStudio. Our current favourite is RStudio. The RStudio desktop version is available via an open-source licence and is free to download and use. You can download the RStudio Desktop IDE from https://posit.co/downloads/.

### 1.1.6.1   *Using an IDE with R (e.g., RStudio)*

If you have installed RStudio and R, then to get started, you simply need to open RStudio (you don't need to open R as well). RStudio presents itself with four windows or panes:

(1) Environment, History and Connection
(2) Source
(3) Files, Plots, Packages, Help, Viewer
(4) Console

You can arrange these in any order you wish by selecting *Tools → Global Options → Pane Layout.*

### 1.1.7   *R as a stand-alone*

To use R as a stand-alone piece of software, click on the desktop icon or select from the list of programs. You should see the graphical user interface (GUI) and a window called the R Console. At the top, there are a limited number of icons and drop-down menus. There is a built-in script editor, and although this is quite basic, you can do everything you need to do using this alone.

The R Console pane is where results or computations are returned. You can type commands directly into the console, but you may find it easier to type commands in the Source pane (RStudio) or in a script (stand-alone R) and submit lines or chunks of code to the console by one of a number of methods (see later).

### 1.1.8 *Launching R*

If you are running Microsoft Windows and assuming that you have not opted out of doing so, the R installer will create a shortcut in the Start menu folder, and you can select the option to create a desktop shortcut. Double-clicking will launch the basic R program. If you are using an IDE such as RStudio, then you do not need to launch R but instead launch the IDE itself (possibly through its own icon).

Using R as a stand-alone (without an IDE), upon starting, you will be faced with the R Console, with a prompt symbol (>). At this prompt, you can enter commands. Start by typing

```
help.start()
```

to bring up a series of manuals and help pages. To see the kind of thing R is particularly good at, type

```
demo(graphics)
```

into the console and hit return, then follow the instructions.

### 1.1.9 *Entering code*

It is possible to execute all commands in R by typing directly into the console and then pressing return, like a calculator. For example, by typing

```
2 + 2

## [1] 4
```

the answer is printed to the console, but nothing is stored. This is an example of an expression command. Expression commands are evaluated and printed to the console. You can recall previous expression commands using the up and down arrows (if you are operating in the console), but to store this value for the future, we need another method.

## 1.1.10  *Reproducing your work*

Whenever we write commands into the console pane and hit return, whatever we have just typed is executed and evaluated by R. This is termed 'executing code on the fly'. While this constitutes a useful means to familiarise yourself with the software or to do simple calculations, in order to perform *reproducible analyses*, you will need some means of recording your work.

To do this, we suggest you type all of your code in a script. In an IDE such as RStudio, a new script will automatically appear in the Source pane when you launch the program – in R (as a stand-alone), it will not. To open a script in R (stand-alone), go to the File menu and select 'New script'. To open a new script in RStudio, do File → New File → R Script or, simply, Ctrl+Shift+N. Either way, you should see a blank page in front of you. Ok, let's create our first script.

## 1.2  Writing your first script

You learn to walk by walking, so what better way to learn to use R than by doing some analysis? We will keep these tentative first steps simple. The analysis is simple, but the results and the implications are profound. We will use a motivating example, one of the most important epidemiological studies of the past 70 years (Doll and Hill, 1964). Along the way, we will introduce some important features of the R language.

Open up a new script file, and on the first line, write

```
# Analysis of Hill and Doll's case-control study
```

## 1.2.1  *Annotating your code*

The hash symbol (#) here is all important. Anything written on the same line after the # and sent to the console is not interpreted by R. This is called commenting. In RStudio, you can comment/ uncomment lines(s) of code using CTRL+SHIFT+C. There are two main reasons to add comments to your script, namely:

- Add remarks to the script file to help remind/inform us what a particular section of code is doing. This is particularly useful if you've had to return to a project that has not been worked on for a while.
- Stop the program from interpreting certain sections of code, you may want to do this when you're working on sections of code but haven't quite finished them yet, or for purposes of debugging.

In the case of the former, it's difficult to have too many annotations in your code, so try to say **why** you are doing something rather than **what** you are doing. Generally, the more, the better. There's nothing worse than having to pick up something you haven't worked on for six months and not recall why you coded something in a particular way, and for what purpose. There is only one commenting code method in R: via the # symbol.

Let's continue. In Doll and Hill's famous study on lung cancer, they sampled cases of lung cancer and matched controls (who were admitted for other reasons) from four hospitals in the UK. It is an early example of a retrospective case-control study. All the important information is contained in just four numbers, or *data points* (see Table 1.1); these are the data we need to enter into R. We will do this by assigning labels to the numbers, thereby creating objects.

### 1.2.1.1 *Assignment*

In order to store and recall numbers so that we can use them again, we need to create an *object* and assign it a value or values. Assignment in R is done using the less-than (<) and dash (-) symbols to create an arrow: <-. An arbitrary number of spaces can be inserted before and after the arrow but not in between < and -. Assignments can also be in the opposite direction (e.g., we could write a <- 1350 or 1350 -> a), but it is more common to do the former. Some people use '=' instead of the arrow, which will work in much the same way but is often considered bad practice. The principal purpose of assigning

**Table 1.1.** The frequency of smokers and non-smokers in lung cancer cases and matched controls (Doll and Hill, 1964).

|  | Cases | Controls | Total |
|---|---|---|---|
| Smoker | $a = 1350$ | $b = 1296$ | $a + b = 2646$ |
| Non-smoker | $c = 7$ | $d = 61$ | $c + d = 68$ |
| Total | $a + c = 1357$ | $b + d = 1357$ | $N = 2714$ |

values as objects is so that we can reuse them in future expressions or assignment commands.

We need to send it to the console to register this line of code and for R to evaluate it. In RStudio, we do this by either placing the cursor on the line you want to submit and pressing `Ctrl` and `Enter` (Windows) or by clicking the Run icon on the top right-hand side of the Source panel. In R, to send a line of code to the console, it is `Ctrl` and `R`. You should see the code represented in the console, but no result is printed. In RStudio, the `a` object should be visible in the Global Environment pane.

### 1.2.2 *Naming objects*

R is case-sensitive. This means the object `a` is not the same as `A`. Many programming languages have official naming conventions, but this is not true with R (Bååth, 2012). Even though there are no official conventions, there are some rules to abide by. Object names can't start with a number but can include underscores or decimal points but not commas, quote marks, or any other symbol, such as `$`, `&`, and `@`. For example, if you wanted to store the value of the 75% centile of some data, you shouldn't call it `75q`, but there is nothing stopping you from calling it `q75`. Above all, try to find the balance between concise and meaningful names; however, recognise that this isn't as easy as it sounds.[4] The data for our example can be entered with the following script:

---

[4]I particularly like this quote attributed to Phil Karlton: 'There are only two hard things in computer science: cache invalidation and naming things'.

```
# Analysis of Hill and Doll's case-control study

# data from the table
# a = No. of smokers amongst lung cancer cases
# b = No. of smokers amongst controls.
# c = No. of non-smoker amongst lung cancer cases
# d = No. of non-smokers amongst controls.

a <- 1350
b <- 1296
c <- 7
d <- 61
```

Finally, be careful of using names that are similar to mathematical constants and the names of common statistical functions. There is only one mathematical constant in common use in R: *pi* is the ratio of the circumference of a circle to its diameter. It is possible to use the name **pi** and assign it a value, so take care in using this. The same applies to function names (we will look at functions in Section 1.4.3). It is possible to give a function you have written the name **mean**, and this will overwrite the existing function. Note that all these changes will only exist in the current session, and starting a new session will revert these functions and constants back to the default setting. We should now save the file, but before we do, let's talk about working directories.

### 1.2.3 *Working directories*

It is worth clarifying what we mean by directories, folders, and *working directories*. A significant amount of pain can be avoided if you understand directories and how to refer to and write to them. It also helps enormously to work within a specific directory when working on data analysis for a particular project. R will, by default, already have a current working directory when you start. To find out what that is, type **getwd()** either in your script (at the top) or directly into the console. This will likely return something like this: [1] "C:/Users/.../Documents", where the '...' will be specific to you and typical for a computer running Windows. This says that R is currently working from the Documents folder of the user named ... within the Users folder of the C drive. This is an example of an absolute directory path that tells R exactly where on your computer you can look for things and save the output. Relative paths (relative to the current working directory) can be used, but specifying the absolute path is a safer option. The advantage of setting the working directory is that you only need to do this once. Any folder/directory can be used, but it often makes sense to create a new folder or directory specifically for your current project.

Suppose you have created a new folder to house your data and syntax for your next analysis project. Assuming you have called it myProject and that it is located in your Documents folder, you will be able to set the current working directory using the setwd() function, with the argument being the name of the absolute directory path,

```
setwd("C:/Users/.../Documents/myProject/")
```

or using the relative path,

```
setwd("~/MyProject")
```

But note that the relative path will only work if the current working directory is "C:/Users/.../Documents/". When the current working directory is anything other than this, the relative path will not work and produce an error – Error in setwd(" /myProject") : cannot change working directory. To save your script file, either press Ctrl + S or go to the File menu. Save the name of the file using the suffix .R. Assuming the file has been saved successfully, you should now see the file's name instead of Untitled1*.

So far, we have only assigned single numerical values to objects; we are now going to enter text data, which will function as labels for the columns and rows of the table.

```
# row labels for the table
rowlab <- c("Smoker","Non-smoker")

# column labels
collab <- c("Cases","Controls")
```

Our label objects each contain two values. To have two or more values in an object, whether numeric or text, we need to use the c() function. The small c stands for 'concatenate', or 'join together'. We can also concatenate objects. For example, we could create an object with the first row of numbers (the smokers) and another that concatenates the second row of numbers (the non-smokers) from the table.

```
smokers <- c(a,b)
nonsmokers <- c(c,d)
```

These two objects, similar to the originals, are examples of vectors; they are of a single dimension – a single row (or line) of values. We now see how to create matrices or *arrays* of values with more than one dimension. We can do this simply by stacking or binding our two existing rows using the rbind() function. For this type of object, we can have row and column names. The row names are inherited from the objects used to construct the table. The column names can be added by using the colnames() function.

```
tab <- rbind(smokers, nonsmokers)
colnames(tab) <- collab
tab

##              Cases Controls
## smokers       1350     1296
## nonsmokers       7       61
```

So far, so good, but we haven't done any analysis yet. To complete our case-control analysis, we are first going to load an external package.

### 1.2.4    *Packages*

Packages are the names given to sets of R functions, compiled code, and sample data. Some are loaded every time you start an R session, and some will need to be installed and added under a directory called 'library' within the R environment. Packages within the system library can be found under the Packages tab in the *Files, Plots and Packages* pane in RStudio (see Figure 1.1). R packages can be installed on your computer (as long as you have an internet connection) from R itself. Once installed, they must be loaded whenever you want to access them. You can install packages in one of two ways: either by typing `install.packages("x")` into the R console or by selecting `Packages`, then `Load Package` from the drop-down menu in stand-alone R, or by clicking on `Packages` from the `Files, Plots, Packages, Help, Viewer` pane in RStudio and clicking install. Try doing this for the package we will use to finish our analysis. First, get yourself to the install packages window (by following the instructions above). Type `epiR` into the box titled `Packages` and click install.

If you are using stand-alone R, select `epiR` from the list (Figure 1.2).

Assuming that the package loaded without errors,[5] there are two options to access functions or datasets from the `epiR` library and any

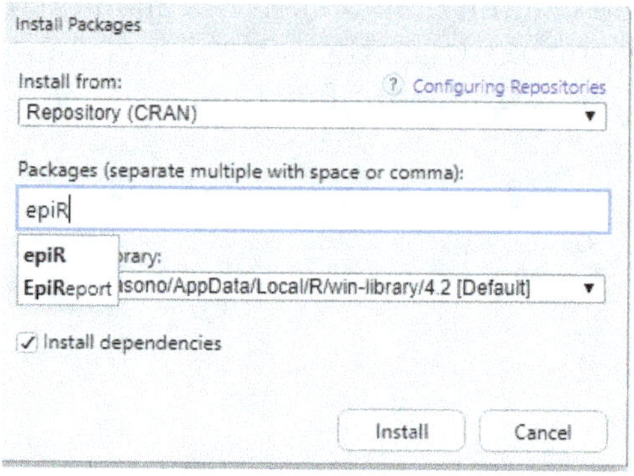

**Fig. 1.1.**   Screenshot of the `Install Packages` window from RStudio.

---

[5]You can check whether the package has been installed by typing `find.package("x")` into the R console.

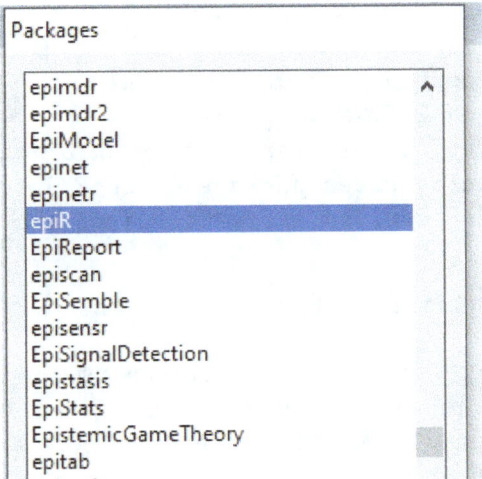

**Fig. 1.2.** Screenshot of `Packages` window from stand-alone R.

package. The first is to use : : in between the name of the package and the function, e.g.,

```
epiR::epi.2by2(tab, method = "case.control")
```

Throughout this book, we use this option mostly to save space. The alternative, and better option if you are to use functions from one package over and over again, is to load a package using the `library()` command, e.g.,

```
library("epiR")
```

You must run the `library()` command for each new session but only install it once. Finally, you can get help on them by typing with `?x` or `help(package = "x")`.[6] To complete our example, we use the `epi.2by2()` function to calculate the odds ratio for these data. We assign the analysis results as an object so that we can use it later and avoid printing too much information to the screen in one go.

---

[6] "x" being a placeholder, of course, for the package you want to load or want help with.

```
library(epiR)
```

```
## Loading required package: survival
## Package epiR 2.0.76 is loaded
## Type help(epi.about) for summary information
## Type browseVignettes(package = 'epiR') to learn how
to use epiR for applied epidemiological analyses
##
```

```
res <- epi.2by2(tab,method = "case.control")
```

Often, many results and the calculations used to derive them are easily accessible to the user for further use. This is one of the great strengths of using R. We can see what has been saved in the **res** object by typing

```
attributes(res)
```

Refer to the help page for the function (in this case, type ?epi.2by2) to know what each specific result refers to. In this example, we want to focus on **massoc.summary**. To do this, we only need to write the names of the object, then a dollar sign ($), and then the name of the attribute we want to access.

```
res$massoc.summary
```

From the output, we can see that the odds of a smoker getting lung cancer are nine times that of the odds of a non-smoker. This output could be redirected to a plain-text file (many other options exist) using the **sink()** function.

```
# create new file called My results- and
# redirect output placed after it to that file

sink("My results.txt")

res

# close the text file
sink()
```

The first few lines of 'my results.txt' look like this

|           | Outcome+ | Outcome- | Total | Odds              |
|-----------|----------|----------|-------|-------------------|
| Exposed + | 1350     | 1296     | 2646  | 1.04 (0.97 to 1.12) |
| Exposed – | 7        | 61       | 68    | 0.11 (0.05 to 0.21) |
| Total     | 1357     | 1357     | 2714  | 1.00 (0.93 to 1.08) |

At the end of a session, save the script file to create a permanent record of your work. When starting a new session, you should be able to 'source' this file (execute all in one go) and reproduce the desired result without further input. This is what we mean by reproducible – we have a record from source data to the result, with all steps annotated, which could be reproduced by someone else.

## 1.2.5 *Environments, objects, and datasets*

When you assign a value to an object in R, R will store the value in the **active** environment under the object's name. The active environment is usually the Global Environment. When you call an object, R will look first in the global environment; if it is not there, it will look along the search path.

```
# A character vector, starting with ".GlobalEnv",
# packages loaded in this session
# then the default packages
# ending with "package:base"

searchpaths()
> searchpaths()
```

```
[1] ".GlobalEnv"
[2] "tools:rstudio"
[3] "C:/Program Files/R/R-4.3.0/library/stats"
[4] "C:/Program Files/R/R-4.3.0/library/graphics"
[5] "C:/Program Files/R/R-4.3.0/library/grDevices"
[6] "C:/Program Files/R/R-4.3.0/library/utils"
[7] "C:/Program Files/R/R-4.3.0/library/datasets"
```

```
[8] "C:/Program Files/R/R-4.3.0/library/methods"
[9] "Autoloads"
[10] "C:/PROGRA~1/R/R-43~1.0/library/base"
```

You can see what is stored in the Global Environment by doing

```
ls(globalenv())
```

or

```
ls()
```

or, when using RStudio, looking at the **Environment** tab in the Environment, History, Connections pane. We suggest storing all of your datasets/databases in the Global Environment (which is done automatically) and not *attaching* a dataset to the R search path using the **attach()** function. Attaching your database means that the database is searched by R when evaluating a variable, and the objects within the database can be accessed by simply giving their names. This sounds convenient but can cause problems when working with multiple datasets/databases. For example, suppose you attach two datasets that have identical names:

```
dt1 <- data.frame(id = 1:5,
age = c(60,55,78,45,83),
sex = c("M","M","F","F","M"))
attach(dt1)
mean(age)
```

```
## [1] 64.2
```

```
dt2 <- data.frame(id = letters[1:3],
age = c(89,95,92))
attach(dt2)
```

```
## The following objects are masked from dt1:
##
##      age, id:
```

```
mean(age)
```

```
## [1] 92
```

While it is convenient to refer to age directly by name, you can probably see that this could lead to confusion when we are working with multiple datasets or objects with the same name. We suggest using `with()` or the $ to access or work within a dataset. For example,

```
with(dt1, mean(age))
```

```
## [1] 64.2
```

```
mean(dt1$age)
```

```
## [1] 64.2
```

```
with(dt2, mean(age))
```

```
## [1] 92
```

```
mean(dt2$age)
```

```
## [1] 92
```

This is less convenient but will make your life easier in the long run.

### 1.2.6 *Masking*

If you load the MASS package and then the dplyr package, you will see the following message:

```
library(MASS)
library(dplyr)

##
## Attaching package: 'dplyr'
## The following object is masked from 'package:MASS':
##
##     select
## The following objects are masked from
'package:stats':
##
##     filter, lag
```

```
## The following objects are masked from 'package:base':
##
##      intersect, setdiff, setequal, union
```

In doing this, you can run into problems if you want to use the `select()` function from the MASS package. R will default to using the `select()` function from the `dplyr` package, as it was loaded last and appears before the MASS package in the search path (see Section 1.2.5). To avoid such problems, you can either switch the order in which libraries are loaded or do the following and write `dplyr::select()` to ensure you have the appropriate function.

## 1.3  Programming with R

### 1.3.1  *Calculation*

We have seen that the R language can function like a calculator. Being a serious piece of software, R evaluates expressions according to BODMAS/BIDMAS (brackets, operators/indices, division, multiplication, addition, and subtraction) rules, e.g.,

```
6 / 2*(1 + 2)
```

```
## [1] 9
```

Dividing by zero yields infinity:

```
1/0
```

```
## [1] Inf
```

Trying to divide 0 by 0 results in 'not a number':

```
0/0
```

```
## [1] NaN
```

R's default behaviour is to print very large or very small numbers in standard form, which is simply a way of writing down very large or very small numbers easily.

```
2^63
```

```
## [1] 9.223372e+18
```

This can be difficult to work with if you are not used to it (or left school long enough ago to forget you were ever taught it); Table 1.2 should help. In summary, for positive integers after the e, move the decimal places that many places to the right; for negative numbers, move the decimal point to the left. Most operators and mathematical functions are as you would expect (see Table 1.3).

**Table 1.2.** Full digit and scientific notation equivalents.

| Full digit representation | Standard form | Scientific notation |
|---|---|---|
| 0.048 | $4.8 \times 10^{-2}$ | 4.8e-02 |
| 0.48 | $4.8 \times 10^{-1}$ | 4.8e-01 |
| 4.8 | $4.8 \times 10^{0}$ | 4.8e+00 |
| 48 | $4.8 \times 10^{1}$ | 4.8e+01 |
| 480 | $4.8 \times 10^{2}$ | 4.8e+02 |
| 4800 | $4.8 \times 10^{3}$ | 4.8e+03 |

**Table 1.3.** Operators and mathematical functions in R.

| Description | R syntax | Description | R syntax |
|---|---|---|---|
| Missing value | NA | Non-real number | NaN |
| Infinity ($\infty$) | Inf | Negative infinity ($\infty$) | -Inf |
| Or | \| | And | & |
| Is equal to | == | Is not equal to | != |
| Equals | = | Assignment | <- |
| Multiply | * | Divide | / |
| Add | + | Subtract | - |
| Modulus | %% | Absolute | abs() |
| Indices (powers) | ^ | Square root | sqrt() |
| Exponential | exp() | Natural log | log() |
| Base 10 log | log10() | Base n log | log(x,base = n) |
| Pi (3.141593) | pi | Factorial (!) | factorial() |
| N choose r | choose() | Relational | >,<=,>= |
| Is distributed as | ~ | List indexing | $ |
| Create a sequence | : | Pipe (magrittr) | %>% |

### 1.3.2  *Floating-point numbers*

It can be surprising that computers do not always compute the correct answer because they might not start with the correct numbers (Thisted, 1988). Look at what happens when we ask R to calculate this simple sum:

```
mySum <- 0.1 + 0.2
mySum
```

```
## [1] 0.3
```

This is what we would expect to see. It should then be true that

```
# == is used to say is "equal to"
mySum == 0.3
```

```
## [1] FALSE
```

Why is it false? Let's ask R for as many decimal places as possible:

```
print(x = mySum, digits = 22)
```

```
## [1] 0.3000000000000000444089
```

Now, we can see the problem. Does this mean R cannot do simple maths? Not exactly. This is not a problem unique to R but to most computer programming languages. Computers don't usually work in base 10 as we tend to; they work in base 2, as it gives the fastest representations. The problem arises because floating-point numbers stored in the computer consist of two parts, an integer and an exponent, to which the base is taken and multiplied by the integer part. In the system used by R, the base is 2, and rational numbers (those that can be represented as a fraction) whose denominator is not a power of 2 cannot be represented exactly. Hence, $1/5$, or 0.2, rounds to

```
print(x = 0.2, digits = 22)
```

```
## [1] 0.2000000000000000111022
```

What we thought were constants (0.2 and 0.1) are approximations to their actual values and, hence, do not precisely match the value of 0.3 when added. For both 0.1 and 0.2 in this example, the closest doubles to 0.1 and 0.2 are larger than the actual numbers. The closest double to 0.3 is a little lower and rounds to

```
print(x = 0.3,digits = 22)

## [1] 0.2999999999999999888978
```

We do not generally need to worry about this, but one problem can arise. It is sometimes necessary to test whether two things agree, and because of floating-point number systems, we will need to avoid doing

```
(0.1 + 0.2 == 0.3)

## [1] FALSE
```

and instead do something like this:

```
mySum = 0.1 + 0.2
tolerance = 1e-10
abs(mySum - 0.3)  < tolerance

## [1] TRUE
```

Or better still, use the **all.equal()** function.

```
all.equal(target = mySum,
current = 0.3,
tolerance = 1e-10)

## [1] TRUE
```

### 1.3.3  *Vectors*

Vectors are the name given to a collection of similar values or data types. Standard vectors consist of numeric values, logical values, or character strings (but not mixed). There are five basic types of vectors: double, integer, logical, character, and complex

(Venables and Ripley, 2000). The two most common numeric classes used in R are integer and double (short for double-precision floating-point numbers). R will automatically convert between the two classes as required, so it is possible to use R without specifying which one you require. Complex numbers are not used routinely in medical statistics, but we provide an example for completeness. Here, we use the function `typeof()` to determine the type or storage mode of an object.

```
vec1 <- c(1,2,3,4,5)
typeof(vec1)

## [1] "double"

vec2 <- c(1L,2L,3L,4L)
typeof(vec2)

## [1] "integer"

vec3 <- c(F,F,F,T)
typeof(vec3)

## [1] "logical"

vec4 <- c("red","blue","green")
typeof(vec4)

## [1] "character"

vec5 <- c(1,2,3) + 0i
typeof(vec5)

## [1] "complex"
```

Scalars (single numbers) can be considered vectors of length one and are not treated differently otherwise. They do not need the `c()` function, but R will not return an error if you do so. Elements of a vector can be accessed or *extracted* by name (if names exist) or by number.

```
x <- c(1,2,3,4)
names(x) <- c("fee","fi","fo","fum")
```

```
# extract the second element of the vector x
x[2]
```

```
## fi
##  2
```

```
# extract the element of x with name 'fo'
x['fo']
```

```
## fo
##  3
```

### 1.3.4 *Vector arithmetic*

In R, you can manipulate numeric vectors in a number of ways. For example,

```
x <- c(2,3,4,5)
y <- c(1,2,3,4)
# multiplication
x * 2
```

```
## [1]  4  6  8 10
```

```
# division
x/2
```

```
## [1] 1.0 1.5 2.0 2.5
```

```
# subtract x from y
x - y
```

```
## [1] 1 1 1 1
```

```
# addition
x + y
```

```
## [1] 3 5 7 9
```

```
# powers
x ^ y
```

```
## [1]   2   9  64 625
```

### 1.3.5 *Extracting elements from vectors*

The : operator is incredibly useful for generating simple patterned vectors and extracting elements from vectors.

```
# a sequence from 1 to 10
x <- 1:10
x

## [1]  1  2  3  4  5  6  7  8  9 10

# extract the 3rd - 6th element.
x[3:6]

## [1] 3 4 5 6

# all but the second element
x[-2]

## [1]  1  3  4  5  6  7  8  9 10

# the first 3
head(x,3)

## [1] 1 2 3

# the last one
tail(x,1)

## [1] 10
```

### 1.3.6 *Character vectors*

Character strings must be entered using matching quotes (either single or double) but will always be returned with double.

```
# a  character vector
colours <- c("green","red","blue")
```

```
# extract the first character of each element.
substr(colours,0,1)
```

```
## [1] "g" "r" "b"
```

```
# alphabet
letters[1:5]
```

```
## [1] "a" "b" "c" "d" "e"
```

```
# make upper case
toupper(colours)
```

```
## [1] "GREEN" "RED"   "BLUE"
```

```
# number of characters
nchar(colours)
```

```
## [1] 5 3 4
```

```
# simple paste example
paste(colours, 1:4, sep = "_")
```

```
## [1] "green_1" "red_2"   "blue_3" "green_4"
```

In this example, we have used the function `substr()` to extract a character vector, the `toupper()` function to turn all elements of a character string into uppercase, and the `paste()` function to concatenate character vectors.

### 1.3.7 *Factors*

A factor is a special type of vector primarily used for categorical data. For these types of data, we use the `factor()` function. For example,

```
bl.type <- factor(x = c("B","B","AB","AB","AB","O","O"))
bl.type
```

```
## [1] B  B  AB AB AB O  O
## Levels: AB B O
```

This is different from a character vector – note the lack of quotations when printed to the console. R internally stores the factor as a set of numbers arranged in alphabetical order relating to the levels.

```
print.default(x = bl.type)

## [1] 2 2 1 1 1 3 3

levels(x = bl.type)

## [1] "AB" "B"  "O"
```

So, in this example, 'B' is stored as 2, 'AB' as 1, and 'O' as 3.

Some categorical variables have a natural ordering. These can be coded using the **ordered()** syntax:

```
y <- ordered(x = c("stage 3","stage 2","stage 5",
"stage 4","stage 2","stage 1"))
y

## [1] stage 3 stage 2 stage 5 stage 4 stage 2 stage 1
## Levels: stage 1 < stage 2 < stage 3 < stage 4 < stage 5
```

But R may not always guess the correct ordering, so we do the following:

```
x <- ordered(x = c("Mid","Hi","Lo","Mid","Lo","Lo","Hi"))
x

## [1] Mid Hi  Lo  Mid Lo  Lo  Hi
## Levels: Hi < Lo < Mid
```

In this case, we should set the levels explicitly.

```
x <- ordered(x = c("Mid","Hi","Lo","Mid","Lo","Lo","Hi"),
levels = c("Lo","Mid","Hi"))
x

## [1] Mid Hi  Lo  Mid Lo  Lo  Hi
## Levels: Lo < Mid < Hi
```

## 1.3.8 *Missing values and other special values*

R uses the symbol NA for missing values. This works well, but a little care is needed if you are dealing with strings that are also 'NA'. On occasion, it will catch you out. For example, if you want to count how many positive, non-missing observations a variable has, you might think that the following would return the correct result:

```
x <- c(1,2,3,NA)
length(x > 0)

## [1] 4
```

However, it doesn't. This is because it returns NA when evaluating whether x > 0. A better way to do this would be to do the following:

```
length(which(x > 0))

## [1] 3
```

'NA' in character strings or names is best avoided. The symbol NaN stands for *not a number* and often arises from calculations that do not make sense or are indeterminate, e.g., 0/0. Negative infinity (-Inf) and positive infinity (Inf) are special values that you may find useful when creating categories from continuous variables, e.g.,

```
x <- c(-1e05,12,15)
cut(x, breaks = c(-Inf,0,Inf))

## [1] (-Inf,0] (0, Inf] (0, Inf]
## Levels: (-Inf,0] (0, Inf]
```

## 1.4 Object types

### 1.4.1 *Matrices and arrays*

It will sometimes be useful to store data not only in vector format (a single column or row of data) but also as arrays or matrices of numbers. A two-way table is a good example:

```
myTable <- array(data = c(59,8,7,26), dim = c(2,2))
myTable
```

```
##           [,1] [,2]
## [1,]       59    7
## [2,]        8   26
```

where **dim** stands for the dimension of the array created using the
**array()** function. Here, we specify two rows and two columns. It is
not limited to two dimensions; normally, two are enough. Note that
elements in the data vector are arranged column-wise in the array
(column-major storage order). A matrix created using the **matrix()**
function is similar but has slightly different arguments; it also permits
row-major storage, e.g.,

```
myTable <- matrix(data = c(59,8,7,26),
nrow = 2, ncol = 2, byrow=T)
myTable
```

```
##           [,1] [,2]
## [1,]       59    8
## [2,]        7   26
```

To extract the elements from arrays or matrices, we simply need
to do

```
X <- array(1:12,c(3,4))
```

```
X
```

```
##           [,1] [,2] [,3] [,4]
## [1,]        1    4    7   10
## [2,]        2    5    8   11
## [3,]        3    6    9   12
```

```
X[1,2] # first row second column
```

```
## [1] 4
```

```
X[,3] # third column
```

```
## [1] 7 8 9

X[c(1,3),2:4] # 1st and third row, columns 2,3,4.

##        [,1] [,2] [,3]
## [1,]    4    7   10
## [2,]    6    9   12
```

### 1.4.2  Data frames

Data frames can be considered a special list type in which all elements are of the same length. They can include different data types, and because of this, they are often used to store datasets. Here is an example using data from a meta-analysis (Gøtzsche and Jørgensen, 2013):

```
# A meta-analysis example.

# Screening for breast cancer with mammography
# Deaths ascribed to breast cancer, 7 years follow-up
# Adequately randomised trials.

event.e <- c(38,38,63,105)
n.e <- c(25214,19711,21088,53884)
event.c <- c(28,39,66,251)
n.c <- c(25216,19694,21195,106956)
adeq <- c(T,T,T,T)
studlab <- c("Canada 1980a","Canada 1980b",
"Malmo 1976","UK age 1991")

dt <- data.frame(event.e, n.e, event.c, n.c,
"adeq rand" = adeq)
row.names(dt) <- studlab

dt
```

```
##                event.e   n.e event.c    n.c adeq.rand
## Canada 1980a       38 25214      28  25216      TRUE
## Canada 1980b       38 19711      39  19694      TRUE
## Malmo 1976         63 21088      66  21195      TRUE
## UK age 1991       105 53884     251 106956      TRUE
```

A few things to note here. We gave names to the rows of the data frame using the `row.names()` function, but we could have just as easily provided study names as a column in the data frame code. We can supply names to the 'columns' of the data frame, but if we don't give a name and instead only list variable names (as we did for `event.e`, `event.c`, `n.e`, and `n.c`), then R will use these names for the data frame. To name a column in a data frame call, use the = operator, as we did with `studlab`. However, note that if you give a name with two or more words and you want to include spaces in the column name, you will need to encase it in double quotes. By default, R then substitutes decimal places for the spaces (as it did here for `"adeq rand"`). Take the hint: R (like other programming languages) does not like spaces in object names! Now, we have created something more complex; we can look at the composition or structure by typing `str()`:

```
str(dt)
```

```
## 'data.frame':        4 obs. of  5 variables:
##  $ event.e  : num  38 38 63 105
##  $ n.e      : num  25214 19711 21088 53884
##  $ event.c  : num  28 39 66 251
##  $ n.c      : num  25216 19694 21195 106956
##  $ adeq.rand: logi  TRUE TRUE TRUE TRUE
```

The output tells us that the `dt` object is of type 'data.frame', with four observations and five variables (or columns). It then reports the variable type of each variable and prints the first set of values (in this case, it is all of them). Before version 4.0, R, by default, converted character strings to `Factor` variables. If you are using a version older than 4.0, then the `studlab` variable will be converted to a factor variable by default. There is an option to convert characters to factors by including an argument in the function statement. We will cover how to do this later in the section on functions.

### 1.4.2.1 *Working with data frames*

Data frames are designed to store datasets or databases in a local environment. You can have as many of these in the current session as your memory will allow. We have previously stated that our preferred strategy for working with R is to work with and within a data frame. We find that using **within()** is useful for doing multiple operations on a data frame in one assignment. The syntax is fairly simple:

```
# a data frame called dt

dt <- within(dt,
{
new.v = x1/x2   # add a new variable
repl = replace(x3, is.na(x3), 0) # replace values in x3
fac  = factor(x4, labels = 1:3) # convert to factor
rm(unused1, temp) # drop 2 columns
}
)
```

Subsetting of rows and columns can be done using the **subset()** function.

```
# filter on vars x1 and x2
subset(dt, x1 == "Low" & x2 < 20)

# select columns (by name or index)
subset(dt, select = 1:3)

# drop columns
subset(dt, select = -(7:9))

# select by column name
subset(dt, select = c("x1","x2"))
```

Adding group averages to a data frame is possible using the **ave()** function; again, use **within()** to add this to the data frame.

```
# to get average of y for each level of a factor or
  group.
dt <- within(dt,{
grp_avg = ave(y, grp)
})
```

Collapsing a data frame can be done using the **aggregate()** function. This is a handy base R function with very general applications. The **by** argument takes a formula-type argument, with the variable(s) you want summarising or aggregating on the left-hand side of the expression and the aggregating factor on the right-hand side of the expression. We demonstrate it here using the built-in dataset **infert**:

```
# get mean age by education
aggregate(infert, by = age ~ education, mean)

##    education       age
## 1    0-5yrs 35.25000
## 2   6-11yrs 32.85000
## 3   12+ yrs 29.72414

# get min age and spontaneous by education
aggregate(infert,
by = cbind(age, spontaneous) ~ education, min)

##    education age spontaneous
## 1    0-5yrs  26           0
## 2   6-11yrs  21           0
## 3   12+ yrs  21           0

# add column new names to first command
aggregate(infert,
by = cbind("mean age" = age) ~ education, mean)

##    education mean age
## 1    0-5yrs 35.25000
## 2   6-11yrs 32.85000
## 3   12+ yrs 29.72414
```

```
# two aggregating factors
aggregate(infert, by = age ~ education + case, median)

##    education case  age
## 1    0-5yrs     0 36.5
## 2   6-11yrs     0 33.0
## 3   12+ yrs     0 29.0
## 4    0-5yrs     1 36.5
## 5   6-11yrs     1 33.0
## 6   12+ yrs     1 29.0
```

### 1.4.3  *Functions*

R has an extensive suite of functions pre-loaded with the base installation, and this can be extended further with a huge range of user-
contributed libraries (see Libraries section). It is also simple for R
users to define their own functions (once you know how). This is,
arguably, what makes R such a powerful statistics software package. We have already met a number of the core internal functions:
`sqrt()`, `factor()`, `ordered()`, and `print()` are all examples of functions. We do not need to know everything about functions in R, but
a little knowledge of how they work will help.

A very general definition of a function is something that takes
inputs and produces an output that is somehow related to the input.
In R, the arguments of the function take the input to the functions
and return the output as a value or values. R functions have named
arguments that can have default values. The `sqrt()` function, for
example, has a single argument (`x`) and returns a single value. The
`data.frame` function has multiple arguments but also returns a single value. So far, we have used functions using 'name = value'. When
we specified `sqrt(x = 40)`, we gave the name `x` as well as the value
40, but we could have directly given the value and omitted the name,
e.g., `sqrt(40)`. This is unlikely to go wrong when there is only one
argument to the function, but for functions with multiple arguments,
there are options. Match the supplied name precisely with the argument name of the function. Hence,

```
sqrt(X = 40)

## Error in sqrt(X = 40): supplied argument name 'X'
does not match 'x'
```

does not work. The **sort()** function has two arguments: **x**, which is the R object to sort, and a logical argument, **decreasing**, specifying whether the object should be sorted in increasing or decreasing order. To call this function with exact matching, we could do

```
x <- c(1,4,2,3)
sort(x = x, decreasing = TRUE)

## [1] 4 3 2 1
```

Partial matching can be done but should be used carefully.

```
sort(x = x, decr = TRUE)

## [1] 4 3 2 1
```

Positional matching is also possible and can be reduce the length of syntax and make code more readable.

```
sort(x,TRUE)

## [1] 4 3 2 1
```

However, positional matching can be vulnerable to errors and if, on updating, changes are made to the argument sequences (Venables and Ripley, 2002). Having unmatched arguments does not induce an error message. For example, the **print()** function has 10 arguments, but it will work when we only supply **x**; the object to print. You can use R without worrying about what the ... argument means in a function, but it would be remiss to ignore it completely. It comes up a lot; for example, it is the first and only argument of the concatenation function (**c()**). In short, it is shorthand for an arbitrary number and variety of arguments, and in the **c()** function, it permits an arbitrary number of things to concatenate. It will also allow arguments to be passed on to other functions, but that is probably more than you need to know at this point. R utilises a range of different naming conventions, so you will come across functions that are all lowercase (e.g., `mean()`, `median()`, and `sd()`), period-separated (e.g., `read.csv()` and `data.frame()`), underscore-separated (e.g., `seq_along()`), lower camel case (e.g., `rowMeans()`), and upper camel case (e.g., `View()`). There are examples of functions with the same name, but one is capitalised while the other is not (c.f. `nrow()` and `NROW()`), with slightly differing behaviours. In some cases, the same name is used by two different packages. Such an example is `select()`. This can lead to the problem of masking.

### 1.4.4   *Working with dates in R*

We often come across dates in our research and need to do calculations with them. A common task would be to calculate the length of follow-up time in survival analysis. There are several ways to code dates in R, and as per our general strategy, we prefer to use the functions in the base R libraries. The trickiest part when working with dates is that they often arrive to you in different formats. They will usually be imported as a character string and need converting to *date* objects. Here is an example:

```
myDate <- "2020-01-01"
```

This is intended to be 1 January 2020. In its current format, the object `myDate` is a character string. We must tell R that we want this to be treated as a date rather than a string. We can do so by using the `as.Date()` function as follows:

```
myDate <- as.Date(myDate)
class(myDate)

## [1] "Date"
```

Once formatted correctly, we can manipulate, add, subtract, etc. For example,

```
myDate + 7

## [1] "2020-01-08"
```

The **as.Date()** function expects the date to be formatted as either *year-month-day* or *year/month/day*. If the dates are in an alternative format, R may not be able to convert it, e.g.,

```
as.Date("1-Jan-2020")

## Error in charToDate(x): character string is not in a
standard unambiguous format
```

In this case, we need to supply the formatting. For this example, this is done by

```
as.Date("1-Jan-2020", format = "%d-%b-%Y")

## [1] "2020-01-01"
```

The date format comprises three parts: letters to represent days, months, and years, each preceded by a %. The separator represents the one used in the date you are trying to convert; these are often '−' or '\' but can sometimes be absent. In that case, you would do

```
as.Date("1Jan2020", format = "%d%b%Y")

## [1] "2020-01-01"
```

where 'd' and 'Y' clearly stand for *day* and *year*, respectively, but 'b' is less obvious – it stands for 'abbreviated month name'. As there are many different permutations of dates, a look-up table is often useful. Table 1.4 can be found by typing **?strptime** but is replicated here for reference.

Base R functions are available to extract parts of date objects: the weekday, month, quarter, or Julian time (days since some origin).

```
d <- as.Date("1973-03-16")   # someones birthday

weekdays(d)

## [1] "Friday"

months(d)

## [1] "March"
```

```
quarters(d)
```

```
## [1] "Q1"
```

```
julian(d)  #Julian Day Number
```

```
## [1] 1170
## attr(,"origin")
## [1] "1970-01-01"
```

Date objects can also be printed to the console or stored in different formats using `format()` (Table 1.5). This function returns the formatted date as a character string, but these could be converted to numeric if required by doing

```
format(d, "%W") # Week of the year
```

```
## [1] "11"
```

```
# or as numeric
as.numeric(format(d, "%W"))
```

```
## [1] 11
```

**Table 1.4.** Table of widely implemented conversion specifications for formatting date objects in R.

| Character | Description | Example |
|-----------|-------------|---------|
| %d | Day of the month as decimal (01–31) | 09 |
| %e | Day of the month as decimal (1–31), no leading digit | 9 |
| %a | Abbreviated weekday name | Wed |
| %A | Full weekday name | Wednesday |
| %b | Abbreviated month name | Jan |
| %B | Full month name | January |
| %m | Month as decimal number (01–12) | 03 |
| %y | Year without century (00–99) | 63 |
| %Y | Year with century | 2022 |
| %H | Hours as decimal number (00–23) | 18 |
| %S | Second as integer (00–61) | 30 |

**Table 1.5.** Output formatting date objects in R.

| Code | Description | Example |
|------|-------------|---------|
| format(d,"%b%y") | Month, year | "Mar73" |
| format(d,"%c") | Date and time | "Fri Mar 16 00:00:00 1973" |
| format(d,"%D") | Month, day, year | "03/16/73" |
| format(d,"%F") | Full year, month, day | "1973-03-16" |
| format(d,"%w") | Weekday as decimal number (0–6, Sunday is 0) | "5" |
| format(d,"%W") | Week of the year (00–53) (Monday as day 1) | "11" |
| format(d,"%C") | Century | "19" |
| format(d,"%R") | Hours and minutes | "00:00" |
| format(d,"%j") | Day of year as decimal number (001–366) | "075" |

There are a number of external libraries which extend the base R range of functions, including data.table, chron, and lubridate.

## 1.5   Loading and saving data

### 1.5.1   *Getting data in and out of R*

Use the load() and save() functions to load and save objects to a specified file (as .RData files), respectively. The function save.image() is a shortcut for 'save my current workspace and all objects within it'. Use dump() to save text representations of the objects on a file. Use the source() function to 'run' a 'dumped' file or any R script.

```
save("x1","x2", "some_objects.RData")

load("some_objects.RData")

dump("x1", "x1.R")

source("x1.R")
```

## 1.5.2 Reading and writing data

A starting point of any data analysis is to input data. There are many ways to do this in R. The first option (assuming that the data are *small*) is to type the data directly to the console or a script. For example,

```
myData <- c(15,18,78,24,13,27,86,61,13,7,6,8)
```

This approach is fine when we have small amounts of data, but more often than not, the data will have many hundreds or thousands of rows and columns, and hence, we will not or should not be typing that in by hand. Instead, we will need to pull data in from another source. This could be a comma-separated file, an Excel spreadsheet, or an exported file from another stats package. Each requires slightly different syntax. For data stored in a comma-separated file (.csv), we would use

```
myCSV <- read.csv(file = "myCSV.csv")
```

where the answer to the argument `file = ""` will be the full directory path where your data file is saved. Note that we have assigned the data as an object with an arbitrary name (`myCSV`), which, although in this case matches the name of the `.csv` file, there is no need for this to match. Reading in Excel files directly requires a package or library to be installed. The future-proof method would be to manually convert the Excel file into a `.csv` file, but this can become laborious and introduces an extra step in which errors could occur. The `readxl` package can read in `.xls` and `.xlsx` files directly. Again, it is assumed that this file is located in your `myProject` folder and the working directory has not changed. We could load this file by doing the following:

```
myExcel <- readxl::read_excel("myExcel.xlsx")
```

For both functions (`read.csv()` and `read_excel()`), R will make certain assumptions as to the form of the data file. For example, `read.csv()` does **not** assume that the file contains the names of the variables as its first line. If your file does, add `header = TRUE`. The `read_excel()` function defaults to reading the first sheet in an Excel spreadsheet, and hence, to read a different worksheet, you can specify either the sheet number or its name using the **sheet** argument.

Plain-text files can be read into R using the **read.table()** function. R can also load data directly from the internet. For either comma-separated or plain-text files, you can give a URL for the filename argument, e.g.,

```
myWebData <- read.csv("http://aWebSite/data/dataset.csv")
```

The **foreign** package has several functions for importing data stored in formats used by other stats packages, e.g., Stata or SPSS. For example, to load in an SPSS dataset (with a .sav extension), we can use **read.spss()**. This function reads a file stored by the SPSS save or export commands. This package also contains functions to read in SAS and Stata version 5–12 binary format files. See https://cran.r-project.org/web/packages/foreign/foreign.pdf for more details on the **foreign** package. To load files in Stata version 13 onwards, you may need an additional package: **readstata13** (see https://cran.r-project.org/web/packages/readstata13/readstata13.pdf. SAS datasets can be imported into R using **read.sas7bdat()** from the **sas7bdat** package. Lastly, it can load Excel files directly from the web. This can prove invaluable when you are performing an analysis that depends on regularly updated data. This approach requires an additional package: **httr()**. The method proceeds as follows. First, obtain the URL and save it as a string object. Then, use the **GET()** function to create a temporary file. It will then be possible to read in the temporary file using **read_excel()** to load it into R. The full code would look something like the following:

```
# A method for an importing excel
# spreadsheet from the web.

library(httr)
url1 <- "https://www.ADataBase.com/cases.xlsx"
GET(url1,
    write_disk(tmp <- tempfile(fileext = ".xlsx")))
myData = read_excel(tmp ,sheet = 1)
```

### 1.5.3 *Recording your work*

R automatically saves a history or *log* file during a session (.RHistory) without a filename prefix in the current working directory. It will save the commands you have sent to the console but not the output. The history can be seen by doing the following:

```
history()
```

To save your own history file, you can do

```
savehistory("myRsession.Rhistory")
```

and retrieve it by doing

```
loadhistory("myRsession.Rhistory")
```

As a tool to help you reproduce your work, using a history file is workable but could be better. For one, it will record all the wrong attempts you made at completing a section of code as well as the correct versions, and it will sometimes take work to track which is which. More importantly, you cannot annotate a file directly with helpful comments and reminders about why you have done something.

## 1.6 Getting help

### 1.6.1 *Internet searches and AI*

It is inevitable that at some point, R will not do as you want or seem to do incomprehensible things. Rest assured, it is not taking a dislike to you; it is only following a set of instructions you give it. Even the most proficient R users will sometimes need help with an error or a confusing result. One of the many advantages of using R is the vast network of online help available. Searching 'how do I do this in R' is often successful. This will nearly always be met with someone who has had the same problem as you and a series of answers from other users with a solution to your issue. At the time of writing, new users are increasingly turning to large language models (LLMs), such as ChatGPT, to find a more comprehensive solution.

## 1.6.2 *Help pages*

Every R function and dataset has a help page. In our experience, they can be difficult for the new user to comprehend, and people often need help deciphering the help pages. This is neither unique to the R language nor the fault of the people writing these (although some are better than others). Most people look at help pages to solve one particular problem. Typically, we would access a help page by using the ? symbol, but this only works if you first know the function names. Let's suppose you want to learn how to do a *t* test in R. You might try

```
?ttest
```

```
## No documentation for 'ttest' in specified
    packages.......
## you could try '??test'
```

You might then try **??ttest**. On this occasion, this is not helpful; neither is **help.search("ttest")**. Doing

```
RSiteSearch("ttest")
```

does bring up some useful links but does not bring the basic *t*-test function to the fore. In this case, addressing your question to a search engine can be quicker. Typing '*t* test in R' is probably the most effective; while not the top hit, the **rdocumentation** page does feature on the first page. Now that we know the function is called **t.test()**, bringing up the help page is simple (e.g., **?t.test**). In doing so, the R Documentation page provides a format for the following sections:

- Description
- Usage
- Arguments
- Details
- Value
- See.Also
- Examples

The description for the **t.test()** is fairly straightforward and states that this function 'Performs one and two sample *t* tests on vectors of data'. The next section, 'Usage', shows the arguments to the function and the order in which they occur, as R syntax. We have two versions for the test: the so-called `Default S3 method:` and the `S3 method for class 'formula'`. This means there are two ways to specify the test: supplying a vector or vectors of data and using a 'formula'. From the Usage section, we can see what (if any) arguments have default answers or values. For example, the argument x has no default value because nothing is written after it. The argument y does default to NULL. The `alternative` argument takes three possible values (`"two.sided"`, `"less"`, `"greater"`). It is the default because `two.sided` is first in this list. The next argument mu is set to zero, and the `paired` and `var.equal` arguments are set to `FALSE`. Next, the arguments are listed in the order they appear, explaining their function and what they control. They tell you what type of input each argument takes. For example, the x argument requires a (non-empty) numeric vector of data values, whereas the argument `alternative` (short for alternative hypothesis) requires a character string giving one of the three possible options. In the `Details` section, specific information about the test is often worth reading before launching into an analysis. The `Value` section lists the outputs that the test returns along with a short description. For the `t.test` function, we can see that calling this function returns a list of class `htest` with 10 components. The `See.also` section provides hyperlinks to similar or related functions. Finally, we have `Examples`, which are often very instructive, as it is often easier to adapt existing code than to start from scratch. It can also be useful to run the example code to see the format of the inputs and to understand more about how the function works.

Aside from `help()`, R has several other functions that can be useful to find help:

- `apropos("foo")`: lists all functions containing the string 'foo'.
- `find("foo")`: lists all packages containing a function called foo().
- `example("foo")`: shows examples of the use of the function foo().
- `RSiteSearch("foo")`: searches for foo in the help manuals and archived mailing lists.
- `vignette()`: shows all available vignettes.
- `vignette("foo")`: shows vignettes for the topic 'foo'.
- `vignette(package = "foo")`: shows available vignettes for the foo package.

### 1.6.3 *Debugging*

Errors in computing are called 'bugs', and the process of removing these errors is called 'debugging'. As you become a more experienced R programmer, you will start writing longer, more complex programs. As with all programming languages, you must always be on the lookout for bugs in your code. Good practice, which includes adding comments, will help you and others navigate around your code, and this will aid in pinpointing bugs as well as improving the transparency of your computer program. If you have bugs in your code, then following these five steps (courtesy of Braun and Murdoch (2007)) may help you find and fix them quickly:

(1) Recognise what type of bug you have.
(2) Make the bug reproducible.
(3) Identify the cause of the bug.
(4) Fix the error and test.
(5) Look for similar errors.

The easiest bugs to fix are those which mean your code does not work at all. Debugging gets harder when the code works but gives 'wrong' answers or, worse, when it only fails for some inputs but not others.

### 1.7 Problems and exercises

(1) Create a vector called `countdown` that is a sequence from 10 to 1 in steps of 1. Then, use the `dump()` function to store the vector as an `.R` file. Load this back into the current R session. Now, save the `countdown` vector using the `save()` function instead. What is the difference between `load()` and `save()` in how they store R objects, and how can they be loaded into the current R session?
(2) Load the built-in dataset `infert` and create a subset that only includes women younger than 40; at the same time, drop the last three columns.
(3) Using the `infert` dataset again, add a new variable that repeats the average age for each combination of the education and case variable. Then, use the `tapply()` function to print the mean age by education and case to the console.

**Table 1.6.** Categories for body mass index (BMI).

| Category | BMI |
|----------|-----|
| Underweight | BMI is less than 18.5 |
| Healthy weight | BMI is between 18.5 and 24.9 |
| Overweight | BMI is between 25 and 29.9 |
| Obesity | BMI is more than 30 |

(4) Enter a vector variable, `weight`, representing the weights (in kg) for five individuals: 72, 84, 61, 70, and 93, and a vector variable, `height`, representing the heights (in m) for the same individuals: 1.76, 1.81, 1.68, 1.79, and 1.83, respectively.

    (a) Calculate the body mass index (BMI) for these individuals and assign the values to a vector, `bmi`.

    (b) Order these individuals' heights according to decreasing BMI values.

    (c) Create a data frame, `mydata`, using the variables `weight`, `height`, and `bmi`.

    (d) Add a factor variable (choosing a suitable name) to the data frame, `mydata`, to represent the categories of BMI in Table 1.6. Check to make sure that the intervals are closed correctly. (*Hint*: check that, for example, a BMI of 25 $kg/m^2$ falls into the overweight category.)

(5) Using the `Sys.Date()` function, print today's date in the day, month, and year format, where day and month are abbreviated and the year is given without century. Use a dash as the separator.

(6) The UKHSA data dashboard is produced by the UK Health Security Agency (UKHSA). The data dashboard was created in response to the COVID-19 pandemic but now contains dashboards of influenza and other respiratory viruses, in addition to COVID-19. Use this resource to complete the following tasks:

    (a) Navigate to the dashboard and download the data for the percentage of people who received a PCR and had at least one positive PCR test result for influenza in the same seven days.

    (b) Load the .csv file into your R session and save it as an object called `influenza_data`.

(c) Determine the number of rows and columns of the data and print out the column names.

(d) Print the first 5 rows of the data to the console.

(e) Determine what type of variable `date` is.

(f) Looking carefully at the format of the data, convert the `date` variable into an R date format.

(g) Sort the data so that the most recent data are at the bottom of the data frame.

(h) Calculate the number of days covered in the data.

# Chapter 2

# Some fundamental statistical concepts in healthcare research

To use R effectively, you will need to know which method to apply and when, and then understand the output R provides; this requires a certain level of understanding of statistics. This chapter and the one that follows provide an overview of the fundamental statistical and key epidemiological concepts used throughout this book.

**Objectives and learning outcomes**

The objectives for this chapter are to:

- introduce different data types and measurement scales
- outline basic ideas of probability and probability distributions
- describe the principles of statistical inference, including estimation, hypothesis testing, and quantifying uncertainty

After reading this chapter, you should be able to:

- calculate simple summary statistics for different types of data
- determine probabilities from probability distributions and select an appropriate probability distribution for use in specific applications
- explain the concept of random sampling, sampling distributions, and estimating parameters of a population
- interpret confidence intervals and the $p$-value for hypothesis testing

## 2.1   What do we mean by statistics?

Statistics is a term used widely throughout healthcare research, but what exactly does it mean? We can think of two ways in which it is used. The term 'statistics' is used to refer to data gathered on birth and death registrations (the so-called vital statistics), but it is also used to mean the practice of 'drawing conclusions from numbers', or, put more formally, the practice of drawing inferences about a population on the basis of observations or *samples*. The word 'statistic' is also used in statistical theory to mean any number that is some function of the data – meaning it can be derived from the data using a mathematical expression.

```r
# some data
x <- c(0,0,0,1,1,1,2,2,3)

# example of a function of x
sum(x)
```

```
## [1] 10
```

```r
# also a statistic, as it is a function of x
sum((x - mean(x))^2)
```

```
## [1] 8.888889
```

When used properly, statistics can help healthcare researchers make sense of data, design better experiments, test hypotheses, and answer important research questions. When used carelessly or for intentionally misleading people, they can cause great harm. Combined with reasoned arguments and credible scientific knowledge, they can be very powerful.

## 2.2   Types of data

We typically start any analysis by looking at what type of data we are dealing with, as this will often determine our approach to analysis.

## 2.2.1  Measurement scales

There are four primary levels of measurement: nominal, ordinal, interval and ratio scale.

### 2.2.1.1  Nominal scales

**Examples:** sex, marital status, blood type, eye colour, and ethnicity.

A nominal scale gives names to a set of mutually exclusive categories. The nominal scale is the weakest level of measurement because you can only group the observations. Frequencies (counts), relative proportions (or percentages), and the modal class are appropriate summary statistics. The mean, median, or standard deviation are not. Pie charts or bar charts can be used to graph nominal scale data. Under certain conditions, the distribution of cases among nominal scale data may be the basis of a hypothesis test (Siegel, 1956).

### 2.2.1.2  Ordinal or ranking scale data

**Examples:** socioeconomic status, income, and Likert scale.

Ordinal scale data gives names to subclasses (or levels) that have a natural ordering, but the differences between subclasses are inconsistent or unknown. The range, or interquartile range, can be used to summarise the variation in ordinal scale data. Pie charts or bar charts can be used to graph ordinal scale data when there is a small number of subclasses.

```
# 1 = Strongly disagree
# 2 = Disagree
# 3 = Neither agree nor disagree
# 4 = Agree
# 5 = Strongly agree

likert <- c(1,2,1,3,5,4,2,3,1,2)
median(likert)
```

```
## [1] 2
```

We should not assume that intervals between adjacent numbers on an ordinal scale are equal. For example, we should not think of 'Agree' to mean twice that of 'Disagree' only that 'Agree' is ranked higher than 'Disagree'.

Ordinal scale variables can be stored as numeric or an ordered factor variable in R.

### 2.2.1.3   *Interval scale data*

**Examples:** Temperature in Celsius or Fahrenheit.

When a measurement scale can be meaningfully ordered, and in addition, the distances between any two numbers on that scale are a known size, the measurement can be considered interval-scaled. In an interval scale, the zero point and the unit of measurement are arbitrary. Interval scale data are truly quantitative (unlike ordinal). As such, all central tendency and variability statistics are appropriate. Scatter plots and histograms can be used on interval-scaled data. Interval-scaled data can be stored using the `numeric()` function as either doubles or integers.

### 2.2.1.4   *Ratio scale*

**Examples:** Temperature in Kelvin, mass, or weight.

When a scale has all the characteristics of interval scale data but also has a true zero point as its origin, it is called a ratio scale (Siegel, 1956). With ratio scale data, the ratio between any two values is independent of the unit of measurement; this is true for weight or mass measured in grams or pounds but not temperature measured in Celsius or Fahrenheit. For example, 100 grams is twice as heavy as 50 grams, and 3.527397 ounces (100 grams) is twice that of 1.7636981 ounces (50 grams) – the ratios are preserved. This is not true for temperatures in Celsius or Fahrenheit; hence, they are interval-scaled. Any statistical test is amenable to ratio scale data under certain conditions. Measurement scales become more descriptive as they progress from nominal to ratio, and more statistical options become available.

### 2.2.1.5 *Overlap of data types*

Data may also be called continuous or categorical. Values of categorical data are often counts of things, whereas continuous data values can, at least theoretically, take any value. Continuous data may appear to be discrete if they have only been recorded up to the nearest whole unit. Age is a good example, as this is often recorded in whole years, but this does not obviate the fact that intermediate values exist and are meaningful.

A continuous variable must be ordinal or interval, but not all interval or ordinal variables are continuous. All nominal data must be categorical. In our experience, many of the measurements used in medical research are ratio-scaled, i.e., they have a meaningful absolute zero. However, it is not uncommon for researchers to *downgrade* ratio scale data to ordinal or nominal by categorising (e.g., '1–4', '5–9', and '10–14') or dichotomising (e.g., into 'high' and 'low'). This is sometimes done to help with interpretation or to meet the assumptions of the statistical tests. Still, often, it is done without an appreciation for what is lost by transforming the data in this way (Senn, 2005; van Smeden, 2022). The researcher will need to decide if the potential loss of information induced by collapsing continuous data into discrete categories leads to a different interpretation.

## 2.3 Summarising data

### 2.3.1 *Categorical data*

When data are categorical, one of the simplest (and often the most effective) ways to summarise them is to count the cases in each category and present them in a table. Here, we use the `apply()` function because the `HairEyeColor` data are in a three-dimensional table.

```
# A count
apply(HairEyeColor,2,sum)

## Brown  Blue Hazel Green
##   220   215    93    64
```

The frequency of green-coloured eyes in these data is 64.

### 2.3.1.1　Frequency distributions

The relative frequency or proportion of eye colour is

```
prop.table(apply(HairEyeColor,2,sum))
```

```
##     Brown      Blue     Hazel     Green
## 0.3716216 0.3631757 0.1570946 0.1081081
```

### 2.3.1.2　Cumulative frequencies

When categorical data have a natural ordering, it makes sense to calculate the cumulative frequency and tabulate the frequencies. The cumulative frequency for a variable's value is the number of individuals or *units* with values less than or equal to that value. The relative cumulative frequency for a value is the proportion in the sample with values less than or equal to that value. An interesting use of cumulative frequencies comes from a study by Croswell *et al.* (2009), in which they report the cumulative risk of receiving at least one false positive result from participating in multi-modal cancer screening. They calculated that, for men, the risk of having at least one false-positive finding was 36.7% (95% CI, 36.2–37.3%) after the fourth screening test (the end of the first day of screening), and 26.2% (95% CI, 25.7–26.8%) for women (see Figure 2.1).

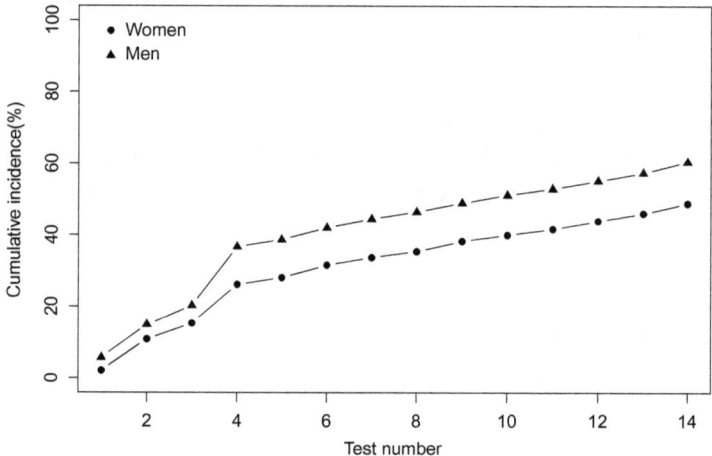

**Fig. 2.1.** Cumulative probability of receiving at least one false-positive screening test for men and women.

The empirical cumulative distribution function can be computed and plotted in R using the `ecdf()` function. The following is an example from Bland (1995), and the data consist of the parity of 125 women attending antenatal clinics at St. George's Hospital.

```
#
parity <- c(0,1,2,3,4,5)
freq <- c(59,44,14,3,4,1)

y <- rep(parity,freq)

cf_fun <- ecdf(y)

# relative cumulative frequency for parity of 1
cf_fun(1)

## [1] 0.824

# plot not run
#plot(cf_fun,verticals = T)
```

### 2.3.2 Continuous data

#### 2.3.2.1 Measures of central tendency

*Means*   The common average or *mean* of any numeric data can be computed in R using the `mean()` function, e.g.,

```
# a vector x with some random data
x <- c(12,65,43,9)

# the arithmetic mean
mean(x)

## [1] 32.25
```

R will default to not removing missing (NA) values before computing the average and so will return NA if any exist. This can be averted using the `na.rm` option, e.g.,

```
x <- c(1,NA,2,3,4,5)
mean(x, na.rm=T)
```

```
## [1] 3
```

```
# or by doing
mean(na.omit(x))
```

```
## [1] 3
```

The mean can be affected dramatically by even a single outlier. The **mean()** function takes an argument **trim**, which is the fraction (0–0.5) of observations to be trimmed from each end of the data vector **x**. We can think of a trimmed mean as an average that is more resilient to outliers. We can think of the median as an extreme form of a trimmed mean – with all but the middle value trimmed!

```
# a vector of length 12, sorted
x <- c(-13,-1,-1,0,1,1,1,1,1,8,12,12)
```

```
# raw mean
mean(x)
```

```
## [1] 1.833333
```

```
# trim 1/12 * 12 = 1 observations from each end.
mean(x, trim = 1/12)
```

```
## [1] 2.3
```

```
# equal to
mean(x[2:11])
```

```
## [1] 2.3
```

There is no geometric mean function in base R or harmonic mean function, but these can be easily coded.

```
# geometric mean
prod(x)^(1/length(x))
```

```
# also the geometric mean
exp(mean(log(x)))
```

```
# harmonic mean
length(x)/sum(1/x)
```

Weighted averages or weighted means are used extensively in meta-analysis. In a weighted mean, each value is assigned a weight corresponding to that value's contribution to the overall average. The arithmetic mean is a weighted average with equal weights. The `weighted.mean()` function allows the user to compute weighted means for a vector $x$, according to a weight vector of the same length.

```
weighted.mean(x = 1:5, w = 1:5/5)
```

```
## [1] 3.666667
```

*Median*    The median is defined as

$$\text{Median} = \begin{cases} \text{the single middle value} \\ \text{the mean of the two middle values} \end{cases}$$

The median of a numeric vector is computed using the `median()` function. Like the `mean()` function, it defaults to including missing values, so if you want to remove missing values, choose `na.rm=T`.

```
y <- c(2,6,7,9,11,15,16)
median(y)
```

```
## [1] 9
```

The median is the 50% percentile or *quantile*.

*Mode* The mode is the value that appears most in a dataset. The function `mode()` does *not* calculate the modal value but returns the storage mode of an object. The mode can often be found by combining `which.max(table(x))`, after checking that a mode does exist and not all values are unique, e.g.,

```
# all unique?
all(table(x)==1)

# find the mode
which.max(table(x))
```

### 2.3.2.2 *Measures of spread*

*Variance and standard deviation* The most common measures of spread or *variation* used in healthcare research are standard deviation (sd) and variance. The standard deviation reflects the scatter about the average, rather than the magnitude of the sample data (Montgomery, 2001). The standard deviation expresses the degree of spread in the original units, and hence when reporting the standard deviation, the units of measurement should be given. This is not true for the variance, which expresses the spread in squared units. There are 'population' and 'sample' versions of standard deviation and variance. The only difference between the two is that the denominator in the sample variance is $n - 1$ and in the population variance it is $n$. R only calculates the sample standard deviation `sd()` and sample variance using the `var()` function. The $n-1$ denominator is used in the sample variance, as it is unbiased for independent identically distributed (i.i.d) data.[1]

```
# the std deviation is the square root of the variance.
sd(x) == sqrt(var(x))

## [1] TRUE

# Population standard deviation in R
# (n in denominator in place of n-1)
```

---

[1]This is true for the variance but not the sample standard deviation (Pawitan, 2001).

```
n <- length(x)
sd(x)*sqrt((n-1)/n)
```

```
## [1] 6.374864
```

If x is an array, matrix, or **data.frame** of continuous variables, **var(x)** will return a covariance matrix with variances on the diagonal and covariances on the off-diagonals.

*Quantiles*   Quantiles are the name given to equal-sized divisions of a distribution. Tertiles divide the data into three equal-sized groups, quartiles into four equal-sized groups, quintiles into five groups, and so on. Divisions into 10 equally sized groups are called deciles.

The **quantile()** function, as the name suggests, calculates sample quantiles of data. It has the following main arguments: **x**, a numeric vector whose sample quantiles are wanted, and **probs**, a vector of probabilities. It also has a **type()** argument for selecting one of the nine quantile algorithms. In this example, the default quantile algorithm (**type = 7**) produces the same result as the **IQR()** function – others do not. It may also mean that R's answers *sometimes* differ from those of Microsoft Excel and other statistics packages. An alternative method for dividing up the data is Tukey's (1977) hinges, which can be found with the **fivenum()** function. These will often coincide with the IQR function but not always. The quartiles are also returned with the **summary()** function.

```
# tertiles
quantile(x, probs = c(1/3,2/3))

# quartiles
quantile(x, probs = c(1/4,2/4,3/4))

# deciles - using the : operator
# to save writing out 1/10, 2/10, 3/10 etc
quantile(x,(1:9)/10)

# Tukey's five-number summaries  = minimum, lower-hinge,
# median, upper-hinge, maximum

fivenum(x)
```

```
# minimum, quartiles, maximum
summary(x)
```

*Range*  The minimum and maximum (the range) of a vector is simply

```
range(x)
```

```
## [1] -13   12
```

The interquartile range (the spread of the middle 50% of the data)
can be found by doing either one of the following:

```
IQR(x)
```

```
## [1] 3
```

```
quantile(x,3/4) - quantile(x,1/4)
```

```
## 75%
##    3
```

*Standardisation and standard scores*  Standard or $z$ scores are the
names given to variables transformed to have zero mean and variance
1. These can be used as test statistics (see the section on significance
tests) and in growth or centile charts. This can be done from first
principles easily enough, but you could also use the **scale()** function
in R. This function was designed to be used on matrices, but it works
for vectors equally as well.

```
# some random data
y <- runif(10, min = 10, max = 20)
#
z <- (y - mean(y))/sd(y)
z[1:3]
```

```
## [1]   1.1458956   0.3868742 -0.8809969
```

```
# or use scale()
zs <- scale(y)
zs[1:3]

## [1]  1.1458956  0.3868742 -0.8809969
```

### 2.3.3    *Transformations*

Many of the methods we use in this book assume that the data come from an approximately normal distribution. Transforming continuous data to satisfy this assumption is standard practice. We may analyse the transformed data rather than the original data and then often back-transform to interpret the results. The most useful transformations in practice are logarithmic, reciprocal, and power transformations, but other options include categorisation or grouping of data (Fig. 2.2). Try log, reciprocal or square root transformations

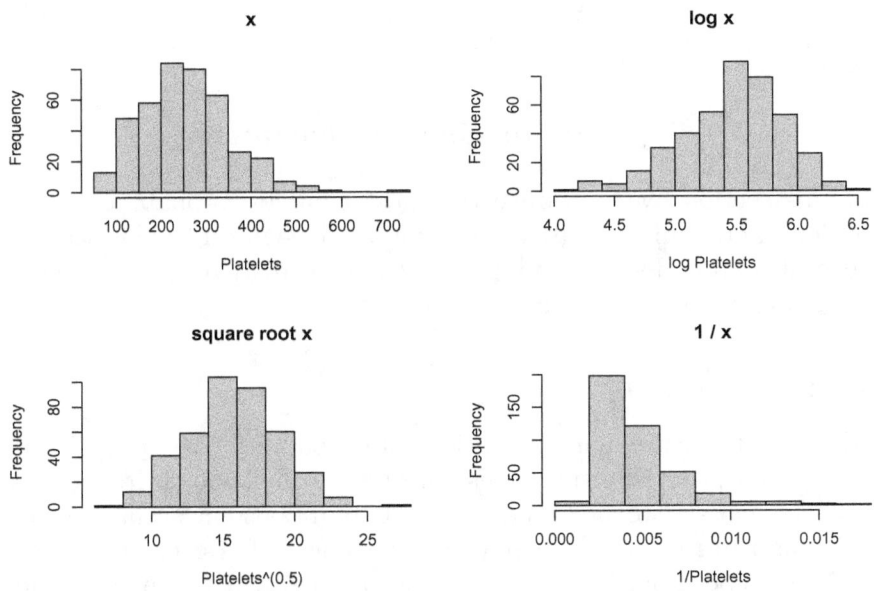

**Fig. 2.2.** Example of log, square root and reciprocal transformations of the `Platelets` variable, in the `pbc` dataset from the `survival` package.

**Table 2.1.** Possible choices for transforming a continuous variable $x$. Adapted from Kirkwood and Sterne (2010).

| Situation | Transformation | R code |
|---|---|---|
| ***Positively skewed distributions*** | | |
| Lognormal | Logarithmic | `y <- log(x)` |
| More skewed than lognormal | Reciprocal | `y <- 1/x` |
| Less skewed than lognormal | Square root | `y <- sqrt(x)` |
| ***Negatively skewed distributions*** | | |
| Moderately skewed | Square | `y <- x^2` |
| More skewed | Cubic | `y <- x^3` |

on positively skewed data, and square or cubic transformations on negatively skewed data (Table 2.1).

The `boxcox()` function in R can be used to find the best transformation of the form

$$u(\lambda) = \begin{cases} (y^\lambda - 1)/\lambda & \lambda \neq 0 \\ \log y & \lambda = 0 \end{cases}$$

## 2.4    Probability and probability distributions

In this section, we introduce the most common probability distributions and some useful R functions for calculating quantiles and generating pseudo-random numbers from the distributions. We start by defining what we mean by probability.

### 2.4.1    *Probability*

Although there are many definitions of probability (see Spiegelhalter *et al.*, 2004), the definition we use throughout this book is frequentist. By 'frequentist', we mean that the probability of some event $A$ equals the long-run relative frequency of occurrences of $A$ over many independent repetitions. Thus, at least theoretically, it requires the idea that the event could be repeated many times. Unlike some other definitions, this definition of probability is rooted in something tangible and could, at least in theory, be empirically verified. This idea is simple to show with statistical simulation.

```
# Simulation of someone tossing a coin
# 10,000 times.
# Assume prob of heads is 0.5
# 0 = tails, 1 = heads

coins <- rbinom(n = 10000, size = 1, prob = 0.5)

# then the long-run frequency should be close to 0.5
sum(coins)/10000

## [1] 0.5078

# Imagine we don't know prob
# use the long-run frequency to estimate prob
coins <- rbinom(n = 10000, size = 1, prob = 0.6)

# estimate p
sum(coins)/10000

## [1] 0.6048
```

Contrast this with probabilities in which repetition makes less sense and cannot be verified, such as the outcomes of elections. We can also determine what data we should expect if the probability was known. For example, assume that the event of a fair coin landing on heads has a probability of 1/2, and from this, we deduce that the relative frequency of heads to the total number of throws of the coin would be equal to or very close to 1/2 over a very large number of repetitions.

### 2.4.1.1 *Some common probability distributions*

There are two broad classes of probability distributions:

- discrete probability distributions
- continuous probability distributions

When a variable is measured on a continuous scale, its probability distribution is continuous. When the variable can only take a limited number of certain values, the probability distribution is called a discrete distribution. The most important discrete distributions are the binomial and Poisson distributions.

The normal distribution is probably the most important distribution in both the theory and application of statistics. The normal distribution is symmetric around the mean, is an unimodal or bell-shaped curve, and is described by two parameters: the mean ($\mu$) and the standard deviation ($\sigma$). The mean gives the location of the central point of the distribution, and the standard deviation determines how spread out the curve is. When a random variable has a true normal distribution, approximately 68% of all values will be between the mean ($\mu$) plus or minus ($\pm$) one standard deviation ($\sigma$), just over 95% between the mean $\pm$ two standard deviations, and 99.7% will be within $\pm$ three standard deviations of the mean. The standard normal is a special case of the normal distribution and has a mean of 0 and a variance (and standard deviation) of 1, often written as $N(0, 1)$. William Sealy Gosset (also known as 'Student') showed in the early 20th century that if the standard deviation is unknown and estimated from a small sample, the resulting distribution is not normal but instead follows a Student's $t$-distribution. Like the normal, the $t$-distribution is symmetric but has a slightly lower, fatter curve than the normal. The larger the sample size, the closer the $t$-curve is to the normal. Unlike the normal, the $t$-distribution depends on the sample size and the degree of freedom. They relate to the amount of independent information left in a sample of data following the estimation of parameters or the calculation of a statistic. Regarding the $t$-distribution, the degrees of freedom are vital in specifying the distribution of the test statistic.

A Bernoulli trial is a name given to an *experiment* or *action* that may result in either of two possible outcomes. Examples include a flip of a coin, the outcome of a binary diagnostic test, or the death of an individual. The binomial distribution is suitable for experiments in which we have a sequence of $n$ independent trials, and the outcome of each trial is either a 'success' or a 'failure'. Assuming that the probability of success $p$ is constant, the number of 'successes' in $n$ Bernoulli trials follows a binomial distribution with parameters $n$ and $p$.

The binomial distribution is a suitable model for comparing the number of times an event occurred and the number of times it did not occur. When this isn't the case, we can use the Poisson distribution. To cite an example from Moroney (1953), if you were to watch a thunderstorm, you could record the number of lightning flashes but not state how many times it did not occur. You can, however, record the time spent observing and then calculate the rate of lightning flashes. The Poisson distribution has one parameter, `lambda`, equivalent to the mean rate.

The exponential distribution is widely used in the analysis of survival or, more generally, time-to-event data. Failure is often used to denote the event of interest in conjunction with the exponential distribution. The exponential distribution has a single parameter: the rate (or $\lambda$), with the mean time to failure given by $1/\lambda$. The distribution is entirely positive, asymmetric, and positively skewed with a long tail.

### 2.4.1.2 *Normal approximation to the Poisson*

As the binomial distribution can be approximated with the normal distribution (Section 2.4.1.3), and since the binomial distribution and Poisson distributions are closely connected, it follows that the Poisson distribution can also be approximated with the normal distribution. If the mean of the Poisson distribution is large (e.g., $\lambda > 15$), then the normal distribution with $\mu = \lambda$ and $\sigma^2 = \lambda$ is a satisfactory approximation (Montgomery, 2001).

### 2.4.1.3 *Normal approximation to the Binomial*

The binomial distribution can be approximated by a normal distribution provided the sample size is large enough and the probability of success ($p$) is not close to 0 or 1. Kirkwood and Sterne (2010) suggest the approximation will hold as long as $n \times p$ and $n \times (1 - p)$ are greater than 10. In practice, this means there should be at least 10 successes and 10 failures. That is, binomial distribution with parameter $n$, $p$ can be approximated by Normal distribution with mean $np$ and variance $np(1 - p)$. See question 8 of the problem and exercise section for an application of this rule.

## 2.4.2 *Working with probabilities and probability distributions in R*

### 2.4.2.1 *Pseudo-random numbers*

Pseudo-random numbers can be generated by computer algorithms. They are not truly random numbers, but have many uses in computational statistics, including simulation, resampling, and estimation. The prefix $r$ is used to denote the functions that can be used to generate pseudo-random numbers in R, e.g., `rexp()` for the exponential distribution. Some examples are

```
# Random numbers from N(0, 1)
rnorm(n = 3)
```

```
## [1] -1.9158871 -0.4583482 -0.9299511
```

```
# Random numbers from N(10, 3.55)
rnorm(n = 2, mean = 10, sd = 3.55)
```

```
## [1] 9.778302 4.559136
```

```
# simulating Bernouilli trials with prob p = 0.2
rbinom(3, size = 1, p = 0.2)
```

```
## [1] 0 0 0
```

```
# simulating 3 Binomial trials each with n = 10, p = 0.4
rbinom(3, size = 10, p = 0.4)
```

```
## [1] 3 4 5
```

```
# Random numbers from exponential distribution with
rate 1/5
rexp(n = 3, rate = 1/5)
```

```
## [1] 2.0554513 3.6970324 0.1885214
```

```
# Random numbers from uniform distribution [0, 1]
runif(3)
```

```
## [1] 0.3518273 0.8075919 0.3109114
```

### 2.4.2.2  *Distribution functions*

The probability distribution function is used to find tail-area probabilities or *areas under the curves* for different distributions (see Figure 2.3 for an example using the normal distribution). It is sometimes called the (empirical) cumulative distribution function, or *cdf* (see Figure 2.4). The prefix p, as in pbinom() or pnorm(), is used to calculate the probability distribution in R. The default is for the function to return $P(X \leq x)$ unless the argument lower.tail=F is used. The distribution function is fundamental to statistics and is used to calculate *p*-values among other important quantities.

```
# Prob that X takes a value greater than +1.96.
# Normal distribution mean 0, sd 1
pnorm(1.96, lower.tail=F)
```

```
## [1] 0.0249979
```

```
1 - pnorm(1.96)
```

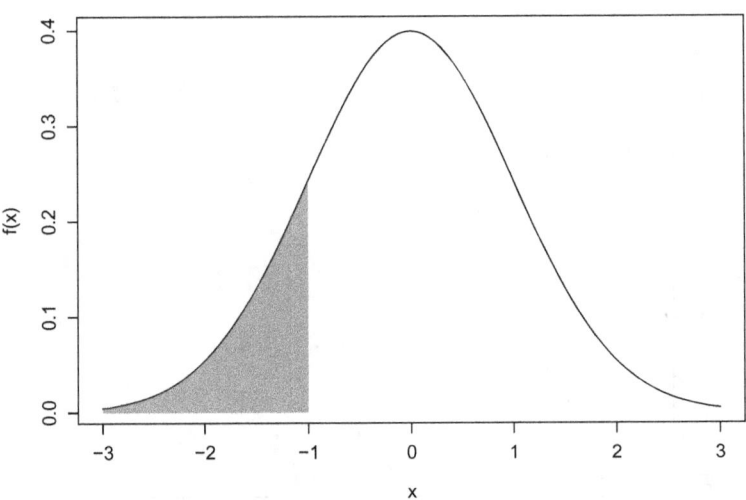

**Fig. 2.3.** Example of a tail area probability for the normal distribution. The shaded region corresponds to $P(X \leq -1)$.

```
## [1] 0.0249979
```

```
# p value for t statistics of 2.56, with n   = 12
(1 - pt(2.56, df = 12-1))*2
```

```
## [1] 0.02651861
```

```
# A non-parametric example
psignrank(19,n=6,F)
```

```
## [1] 0.03125
```

```
# P(a < X <= b) - area of an interval.
# Example using Poisson distribution.
a <- 3
b <- 4
ppois(b,lambda = 1) - ppois(a, lambda = 1)
```

```
## [1] 0.01532831
```

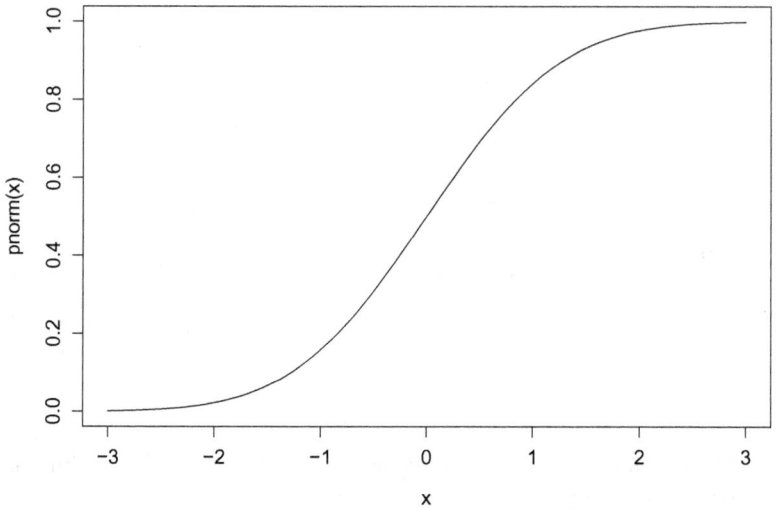

**Fig. 2.4.** Cumulative distribution function for the normal distribution.

### 2.4.2.3 *Quantile function*

The quantile function returns the value of a random variable such that it makes the probability less than or equal to a specified probability. It is sometimes referred to as the inverse cumulative distribution function and may help to think of this function as reversing the operation of the cumulative distribution function. It is used in statistics to find critical values for statistical tests, among other uses. The prefix for quantile functions in R is q, as in qnorm()

```
# critical value for a t test
# with 6 degrees of freedom
# and significance level 0.05

alpha <- 0.05
qt(1 - alpha/2, df = 6)

## [1] 2.446912

# Critical value for the 2-way table
qchisq(1 - alpha, df  = 1)

## [1] 3.841459
```

### 2.4.2.4 *Density functions*

If a probability distribution is discrete (takes only integer values), then the probability density function (pdf) returns the probability that a random variable $X$ takes the value $x$, written $P(X = x)$. If the probability distribution is continuous, then the density function returns the gradient of the slope of the cumulative distribution function at $x$; see Figure 2.4. In R, density distribution functions follow a convention of the letter $d$ followed by the name of the distribution, e.g., dnorm().

```
# probability of getting 6 heads
# in 10 throws of a fair dice
dbinom(6, 10, 0.5)

## [1] 0.2050781

# probability of exactly 1 bus
# arrives if they arrive on average
```

```
# every seven minutes
dpois(1,7/60)
```

```
## [1] 0.1038195
```

```
# Gradient of the exponential cdf with
# mean of 2 years, at value x = 5 years
dexp(5,1/2)
```

```
## [1] 0.0410425
```

## 2.5    Sampling, significance tests, and confidence intervals

### 2.5.1    *Why do we sample?*

In any research setting, there will often be limits on resources (money, time, and effort), accessibility, and utility (Barnett, 1981). Even if we had the resources to do it, it could be unethical to subject the whole population to some intervention or experimental drug. We often aim to minimise the sample size while maintaining a reasonable chance of success. There are diminishing gains as the sample size increases, whilst costs usually increase linearly. Occasionally, we might have access to the whole population – vital statistics such as births and deaths often capture the entire population at any one time. Still, most often, we work with samples rather than populations.

### 2.5.2    *Sampling distributions*

The following code simulates the process of sampling from a population:

```
true.mean <- 65
true.sd <- 4.472
n <- 20

# simulate a population of arbitrary size
P <- rnorm(10000, true.mean, true.sd)
```

```
# this is a one random sample from it
set.seed(111)
sample1 <- sample(x = P, size = n,T)
sample1[1:3]
```

```
## [1] 67.48671 72.90424 60.72899
```

```
mean(sample1)
```

```
## [1] 64.9497
```

```
# this is another sample from
sample2 <- sample(x = P, size = n,T)
mean(sample2)
```

```
## [1] 66.63348
```

From this, we can see that the mean of a random sample will vary. If we replicated this sampling over and over again, we could collate all the sample means into a distribution: a sampling distribution. Statistical theory tells us what this distribution looks like – what the centre of this distribution is and how spread out it will be. We know that if the sample is random, then the average of the sampling distribution will be equal to the population average, and the standard deviation of the sampling distribution will be the population's standard deviation divided by the square root of the sample size $n$. We will also see in a later section that under very broad conditions, the shape of the sampling distribution will be normal. The following code provides a demonstration of this:

```
# this code replicates the sampling process used above
# doing it 1000 times
# and stores the mean - forming a sampling distribution.
rs <- replicate(1000, mean(sample(x = P, size = n, T)))

# mean of the sampling distribution
mean(rs)
```

```
## [1] 65.07732
```

```
# std dev of the sampling distribution
(std.err <- sd(rs))
```

```
## [1] 1.019454
```

```
# close to
(true.std.err <- true.sd/sqrt(n))
```

```
## [1] 0.9999696
```

### 2.5.2.1   Standard error

The standard deviation of the sampling distribution gets its own name: the standard error. The standard error measures how far from the population value the sample estimate is likely to be in any sample. It is also seen as a measure of statistical accuracy (Efron and Tibshirani, 1994) because the smaller it is, the closer to the truth you are likely to be in any one sample. Using the properties of the normal distribution, in the long run, 67% of sample means will be within $\pm 1$ standard error of the population mean, and 95% will be within $\pm 1.96$ (or approximately 2) standard errors.

Another important result builds on this idea: the confidence interval. When the population distribution is normal and the sampling is random, 95% of the sample means will be within $\pm 1.96$ standard errors; it must also be true that an interval centred around the sample mean and extending out to 1.96 standard errors must contain the true mean 95% of the time.

This idea is the basis for the confidence interval, which says that an interval based on the sample mean $\pm 1.96$ standard errors will contain the true mean 95% of the time under certain conditions.

### 2.5.2.2   Central limit theorem

The central limit theorem (CLT) is arguably the most important theorem in statistics. The theorem states that the sum of $n$ *independent* random variables will follow an approximate normal distribution (Gelman and Hill, 2007). The approximation improves as $n$ increases. In many cases, the approximation will be good for small $n$, but in some cases, we may require a very large $n$ (in the hundreds) for the approximation to be satisfactory. In general, if the random variables are identically distributed, and the distribution of each one does not

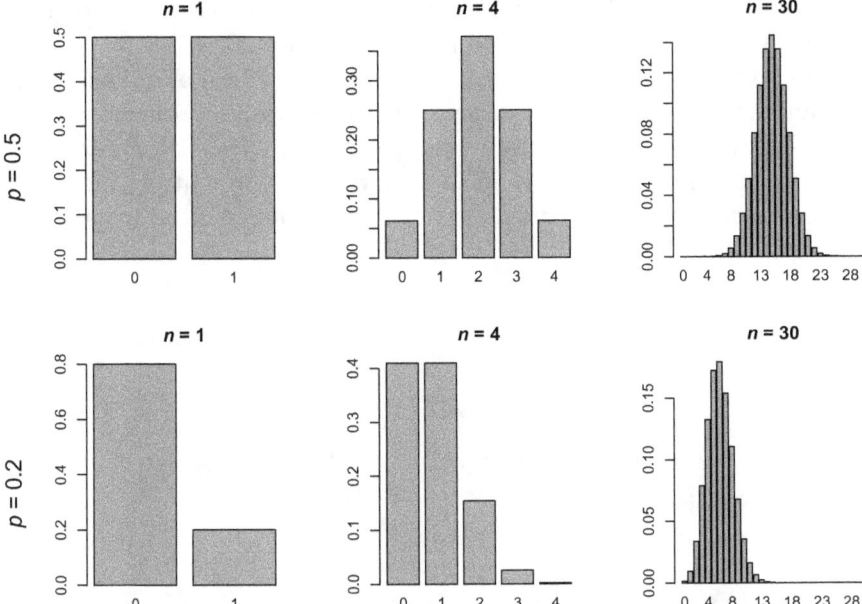

**Fig. 2.5.** Illustration of the central limit theorem (CLT) using the sum of independent binomial random variables each with $p = 0.5$ (top panel) and $p = 0.2$ (bottom panel).

depart radically from the normal, then the central limit theorem works reasonably well, even for $n = 4$ (Montgomery, 2001).

Figure 2.5 shows how the CLT works, starting with a single toss of a coin and the outcome of the number of heads. For one throw of the coin, the probability distribution is uniform (and definitely not normal); however, as we move to more than one throw of a coin to $n = 4$, $n = 10$, and then $n = 30$, the distribution tends to be normal as predicted. The speed (in terms of $n$) at which this happens varies, but the theorem holds under a wide range of conditions.

### 2.5.3 Confidence intervals

When we taught confidence intervals to undergraduate medical students in Oxford, we would ask each student (in eight small classes, each with 20–25 students) to draw a set of 12 numbers from a much more extensive list for which the mean was known to us but not

revealed to them. We instructed the students to use a die to select
the 12 numbers from the list to mimic a random draw. Each student
would then calculate the sample mean and a 95% confidence interval and was then invited to come up to the front. From experience
and theory, we knew that we were guaranteed to get the majority of
these confidence intervals (~95%) to cover the 'population' mean and
a small percentage that would not. The following R code recreates
the class experiment:

```
data(LVD, package = "R4HCR")

# population is 144 individuals arranged in 4 blocks
# sampling is done with two dice -
# scores indicate which row and column to select
# sample, three from each of the four blocks
# sample size n = 12

# simulate 12 throws of 2 die
die1 <- sample(x = 1:6, 12, T)
die2 <- sample(x = 1:6, 12, T)

# drawing the numbers from the blocks
smp <- c(
LVD[[1]][cbind(die1[1:3],die2[1:3])],
LVD[[2]][cbind(die1[4:6],die2[4:6])],
LVD[[3]][cbind(die1[7:9],die2[7:9])],
LVD[[4]][cbind(die1[10:12],die2[10:12])]
)

# the first four numbers of our sample
smp[1:4]

## [1] 5.48 5.04 4.03 4.73
```

In Figure 2.6, of the 25 intervals calculated, two lie completely
outside the true mean, which is entirely consistent with the theory. If
we were to consider all of the intervals calculated in all the sessions we

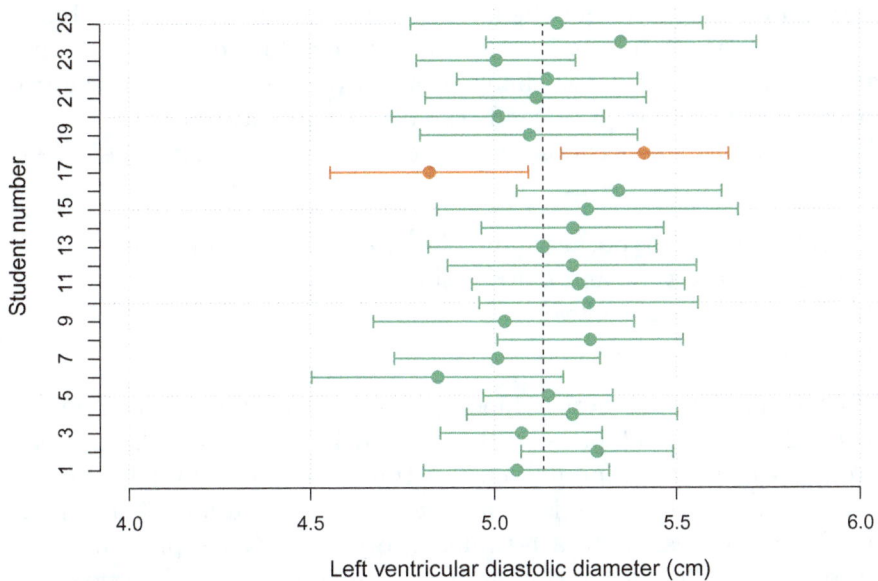

**Fig. 2.6.** A simulation of the class sampling experiment with 25 confidence intervals calculated from $n = 12$.

have taught, the number of intervals that included the mean would be very close to 95%. In everyday situations, we will, of course, calculate only one confidence interval, and although we cannot guarantee that it will not be the one that doesn't contain the true mean, given what you have just seen, would you be willing to bet a significant sum of money that it doesn't?

### 2.5.4 *Tests of significance*

The majority of statistical analyses in healthcare research involve comparison between treatments (or procedures) or between groups. For example, suppose an experimental drug was given to people to see if it lowered their blood pressure. The null hypothesis states that the drug has no effect on the blood pressure: the blood pressure is the same before and after taking the drug. One possible alternative hypothesis is that the drug lowers blood pressure. An experiment to test this hypothesis is conducted. A number or patients are recruited and randomised to either the new treatment or a placebo. The blood pressure of the patients is measured at the start of the study and at the end to see if it has changed. The averages changes in the two groups are then compared and tested using a statistical test.

In general, when choosing a statistical test for hypothesis testing, we

1. state the null hypothesis and the alternative hypothesis
2. consider the type and distribution of measurements
3. choose significance level
4. compute a $p$-value.

Suppose in our hypothetical blood pressure trial, the treatment group lowered their blood pressure by 5 mmHg more than the placebo group. We would want to know if this difference could be due to chance or whether this is more likely to be a result of the drug. To do this we calculate a $p$-value. The $p$-value is the probability of observing a difference of this size (or bigger) if the drug had no effect on blood pressure. If the probability is small then a difference of this size is unlikely under the null hypothesis and evidence against the null hypothesis. Conventionally, we use a significance level of 0.05 but $p$ values of 0.01 are also used. Suppose that in our hypothetical example, the $p$-value we calculate is 0.015. This would tell us that difference observed between the groups is unlikely to have occurred if the drug really didn't work and so we would reject the null hypothesis, and conclude there is evidence that drug can lower blood pressure.

### 2.5.5   *The p-value*

The $p$-value tells us how likely the data (or more extreme) will occur were the null hypothesis true. It is interpreted as a measure of the implausibility of the observations obtained in an experiment and the strength of evidence against the null hypothesis. How do we decide what is strong enough evidence against the null hypothesis? Conventionally, we consider a statistical significance level of 5% as the threshold in medical science. Although widely used throughout science, there are a number of common misconceptions held about the $p$-value.

- *The p-value is the probability that the null hypothesis is true.* The p-value is <u>not</u> the probability that the null hypothesis is true. A p-value of 0.05 does not mean there is a 5% probability that the null hypothesis is true. This is a common misconception and should be avoided.
- *A non-significant difference (e.g., $p > 0.05$) means there is no difference.* A non-significant result may arise simply because the study was not capable of detecting it (e.g., the sample size was too small). A non-significant p-value means that the observed results are consistent with a 'null' effect but are also consistent with the range of effect sizes spanned by the confidence interval. This is sometimes summarised as 'absence of evidence is not evidence of absence'.
- *'Statistically significant' findings are clinically important.* The p-value does not tell you about the magnitude of the effect. When the sample size is large, it is quite common to find statistically significant results that are of little clinical consequence. Consult with a specialist to determine the clinical importance of the finding and don't rely solely on the p-value.
- *An important difference exists between a p-value of 0.049 and a p-value of 0.051.* The problem with setting a threshold for interpreting p-values (in this case, 0.05) is that it creates an artificial distinction between results that fall closely on either side of this dividing line. Regarding the strength of evidence, there is very little difference between p-values of 0.051 and 0.049.

### 2.5.6    *Hypothesis testing and hypothesis generation*

It is important to recognise the difference between hypothesis testing and hypothesis generation. The statistical procedures are the same, but the interpretation of results is quite different. If you closely examine any dataset, you will likely see patterns that, in retrospect, might appear unlikely to have arisen by chance. By definition, one in 20 tests we carry out at the 5% significance will be 'statistically significant' even if when there are no real differences. Suppose we see unanticipated patterns in a dataset that appear unlikely to have arisen by chance. In that case, we have generated a new hypothesis that needs to be tested on a new dataset – you cannot test a hypothesis on the same data that generated it. To have any credibility, the

hypotheses to be tested must be pre-specified in the research proto-
col. However, we do not wish to prevent researchers from carrying
out meticulous exploratory data analyses as this can be highly pro-
ductive but only to warn against the very real threat of being misled
by randomness.

### 2.5.7 *Analysis of variance*

The analysis of variance (ANOVA) is used for several analyses in
this book, including the calculation of the intra-class correlation and
measurement error. ANOVA has many wide-ranging applications in
statistics, and a complete introduction to the subject is beyond the
scope of the book. Briefly, the ANOVA compares different sources of
variation to test a hypothesis about averages. We demonstrate this
using a simple example.

#### 2.5.7.1 *Example: Comparing the effect of low, medium, and high doses of a treatment*

Consider an experiment in which 12 individuals are assigned randomly to a treatment given at low, medium, or high doses. Some
measure of response is taken shortly after administration of the therapy; see Table 2.2.

**Table 2.2.** Results of a hypothetical experiment in which there are four replicate measurements for three doses of a treatment.

| | Dose | |
|---|---|---|
| Low | Medium | High |
| 4 | 6 | 8 |
| 5 | 6 | 6 |
| 5 | 8 | 12 |
| 6 | 9 | 9 |
| $\bar{y}_1 = 5$ | $\bar{y}_2 = 7.25$ | $\bar{y}_3 = 8.75$ |
| | $\bar{y} = 7$ | |

An ANOVA table generated using R looks like this

```
## Analysis of Variance Table
##
## Response: y
##           Df Sum Sq Mean Sq F value  Pr(>F)
## dose       2   28.5 14.2500  4.6636 0.04075
## Residuals  9   27.5  3.0556
```

The ANOVA table shows how the total variability of data is partitioned into variability between the group averages, and variation between individuals within each group. As the null hypothesis is that the group averages are equal, the ratio of the variation within-groups to between groups is also expected to be equal. The null hypothesis can be rejected if the variance between groups is much larger than the within-group variances. The ANOVA table in our example, has rows labelled **dose** and **Residuals**. The row labelled dose corresponds to the variability of the low, medium and high dose group averages (5, 7.25, and 8.75) and the row labelled **Residuals** corresponds the variability within the dose groups (e.g., the 4, 5, 5, 6 in the low dose). The ANOVA table provides a way to compare the two sources of variability on a common scale – the mean square. We can see from the ANOVA output that the mean square for the dose group averages is 14.25. The mean square for within-groups is 3.0556. The mean square between groups is 4.66 times of the mean square within groups. The ratio of the two mean squares is called the $F$ value and this can be compared to a reference $F$ distribution, and a $p$-value calculated. The $p$-value of 0.04075 provides evidence to suggest the variability seen between the groups is larger than we would expect by chance. We could conclude that the doses produce different responses.

## 2.5.8   *Non-parametric methods*

Some statistical tests assume the measurement data are drawn from a probability distribution (e.g., normal distribution). Still, other methods do not require these types of assumptions – they are called non-parametric methods. Most operate by converting the measurement data into ranks or signs (e.g., Wilcoxon rank sum and log-rank test). These tests have fewer assumptions but are considered less powerful than parametric tests and, for that reason, are seen as a second choice to the parametric equivalents. The performance of these tests can also be impaired when the data are tied.

### 2.5.9   *Statistical modelling*

Statistical modelling is a term used to describe the process of developing and fitting statistical models to data. They are typically off-the-shelf models that are general enough to be applied to a wide range of settings. They often explain the relationships between many variables using only a few parameters, although some machine learning models can have hundreds or thousands of parameters. Models have many practical uses and are used widely in medical research. They are often used to analyse clinical trial results, find important correlates of diseases, assist clinicians with diagnosis and predict the risk of future health outcomes. For example, in the UK, a patients' 10-year risk of developing conditions like heart attack, stroke, and other cardiovascular disease is calculated using an equation developed from a statistical model. Clinical prediction models such as these, are now used throughout medicine and can help health professionals make more evidence-based decisions.

### 2.5.10   *Assumptions*

All of the tests and models described in this book have assumptions – things we must assume to be true for the method or test to have the properties they claim. In this book, we encourage the reader to check the assumptions before applying the test or model and to test these assumptions objectively where possible. In each example, we will specify which assumptions are required for each analysis. Many models and tests share the same assumptions, so it is expedient to list them here and then refer to them in each individual case.

#### 2.5.10.1   *Assumptions common to all analyses*

The following assumptions apply to all of the methods described in this book.

*A0 Representativeness. The samples should be representative of the target population.* This is satisfied with *true* random sampling. With random sampling, the only way the sample can differ from the population will be due to chance. Statistical analyses are frequently conducted on the assumption that the samples are random. This is, in fact, rarely the case, as a truly random sample (where each member of a population has an equal chance of being sampled) is seldom feasible or practical. Instead, samples are chosen for convenience and ease of access. Sometimes, the sample is based on the experimenter's intuition or judgement, which can be sufficient, but this is subjective and may lead to an unrepresentative sample. Although this standard is rarely met, it does not mean we cannot produce robust conclusions from data, but we must always reflect back on how the data were collected or sampled, identify to whom the results generalise, and identify any potential systematic biases.

*A1 Mutual independence. The samples (within groups) are not linked or related in any sense.* All of the statistical methods in this book assume that the observations are mutually independent. In other words, the value of any one observation is not linked to that of another. Mutual independence is usually satisfied when the outcomes are measured on unrelated members or *units*. The most obvious violation of this is when multiple measurements are taken on the same individual. This type of pseudo-replication tends to overstate the amount of data there is and leads to spurious precision. Milder forms of non-independence occur when there are clusters or structures, which means specific adjacent samples are more similar to each other than non-adjacent data points. We will also need to consider independence between groups when running some tests, such as the *t* test.

### 2.5.10.2 *Assumptions specific to certain methods*

The following represent assumptions that may only be relevant for some methods and tests.

*A2 Independent groups. The members of the groups being compared are independent of each other.* If the two groups or *samples* are made up of entirely different members, then A2 is most likely satisfied. If the two groups are instead composed of the same participants measured *before* or *after* some intervention, we would assume that they are not independent.

*A3 Normality. The outcomes* $Y_i, \ldots, Y_n$, *or residuals* $\epsilon_i, \ldots, \epsilon_n$ *are approximately normally distributed.* Many of the methods we use in this book assume that either the outcome or the residuals (the difference between the expected values and the observed) are approximately normally distributed. When there are sufficient data, this assumption can and should be checked. Gross deviations from normality should be addressed either through transformation or by using a method that does not make this assumption.

*A4 Equal variances. The residuals have constant variance.* The analysis of variance has an assumption that the variances of the groups being compared are equal. This assumption can be tested using an $F$ test.

*A5 Bivariate linearity: Two variables, X and Y, have a linear relationship.* This assumption is relevant when we consider measuring the strength of association with correlation coefficients or simple linear regression.

*A6 Monotonicity: The relationship between X and Y is either entirely non-increasing or entirely non-decreasing – it does not change direction.* This assumption is relevant when we consider measuring the strength of association with correlation coefficients.

## 2.6 Problems and exercises

(1) Load the `lung` dataset from the `survival` package and complete the following tasks.
   (a) Obtain summary statistics (min, mean, median, etc.) for all of the variables in the dataset. What are the median and range of the age of the participants?
   (b) Find the median survival time in those with `status==2`.
   (c) The `lapply()` and `sapply()` functions allow you to apply a function over a list or vector. Use lapply to obtain the median for all of the variables in the `lung` dataset.
   (d) Adapt the `lapply` expression above to ignore missing values.

(e) Now, use the `sapply()` function to do this; what is the difference?

(f) Both `lapply` and `sapply()` accept user-defined functions of the form `function(x)f(x)`, where `f(x)` is some function of `x`. Use either `lapply` or `sapply` to sum the number of missing values across all variables in the dataset.

(2) Continue with the `lung` dataset:

(a) Add a factor variable `agegroup` which divides patients into four age groups (younger than 55, 55–64, 65–69, and 70 or older).

(b) Convert the `sex` and `status` variables into factor variables and label the `sex` variable 'female' or 'male', and the `status` variable as 'censored' or 'dead'. Refer to the help page to make sure you apply the labels correctly.

(c) What is the percentage of male participants?

(d) Use the `xtabs()` function to produce a cross-table of age group and status.

(e) Produce a table that gives the mean age for each age group.

(f) Produce a data frame containing the median follow-up time according to patients alive or dead at the last contact (*Hint*: use `aggregate()`). Provide an informative label for the column with the median time.

(g) What type of variable is `ph.ecog`. Find the modal value of this variable, giving the answer in terms of the clinical label rather than the numerical score.

(h) Calculate the empirical cumulative distribution function of the `ph.ecog` variable and use this function to calculate the relative cumulative frequency of patients with a ph.ecog score $<= 2$ (*Hint*: use the `ecdf()` function).

(i) Log-transform the survival time (in days) variable and then find the geometric mean. Compare this value with the mean of the untransformed survival time.

(3) A radiologist is asked to give her confidence in whether a lesion on a CT scan is malignant in a score of 0–100. What type of measurement scale is this and why? What kind of data summaries would be appropriate for these data?

(4) Is the Poisson distribution an example of a continuous or discrete probability distribution?

(5) Find the mean and standard deviation of a normal distribution that could be used to approximate a Poisson distribution with $\lambda = 30$. Use the `rpois()` function and compare the quantiles from the simulated data to those from a true normal distribution.

(6) What is the probability that of $n = 10$ births, exactly nine will be female, assuming the probability of a male birth is 0.5?

(7) What is the probability that of $n = 30$ births, there will be fewer than or equal to 10 male births?

(8) The birth sex ratio in the UK in 2020 was approximately $105 : 100$; that is, there were on average 105 male births for 100 females births. Describe a probability distribution that could approximate the birth sex probabilities, stating the parameters of the model.

(9) For a single sample $t$ test, the degrees of freedom are equal to $n - 1$. Find the multiplier for a confidence interval for a sample of $n = 12$ and a significance level of $\alpha = 0.05$.

(10) Find the probability value that corresponds to a $t$-statistic of value 2.109816 obtained from a sample of size $n = 18$.

(11) Suppose, under normal conditions, the fraction of defective medical devices in a manufacturing setting is $1/100$. What number of defectives in a batch of 50 would suggest that the process is out of control and producing too many defective items. Assume a probability of less than 1% is evidence that the process is out of control.

(12) Table 2.3 shows the cumulative rate of false positive screens (Croswell *et al.*, 2009). Using a Poisson distribution, approximate the number of false positive results. First, determine the average number of false positive results, and then use the density function to assess the goodness of fit.

**Table 2.3.** Number of people with one or more false-positive result (38919 had no false positives).

| 1 | 2 | 3 | 4 | 5 | 6 | 7 | ... | > 10 |
|---|---|---|---|---|---|---|-----|------|
| 18394 | 6043 | 2531 | 1535 | 642 | 228 | 78 | ... | 0 |

(13) Under the exponential distribution, the probability that a patient fails before the average time is $p = 0.63$, which is true regardless of what the rate of events is (Montgomery, 2001). Using the appropriate functions, show that this is true for an arbitrary rate.

(14) The $\chi^2$ probability distribution with $n$ degrees of freedom has a mean equal to $n$ and a variance equal to $2n$. Using pseudo-random numbers, show that this is true if the sample of random numbers is large enough.

(15) Table 2.2 showed the results of a hypothetical experiment in which there are four replicate measurements for three doses of a treatment. Using the data in the table and the ANOVA output, answer the following questions

   (a) Show that the sum of squares due to dose is equal to the variance in the group averages multiplied by the degrees of freedom for dose and the number of replicates.

   (b) Calculate the $p$-value shown in the ANOVA table using the pf() function.

(16) Find the critical value for a signed rank test with 15 observations and a significance level of 0.01.

# Chapter 3

# Measures of disease occurrence

In this chapter, we describe some key concepts and measures of effect used in healthcare research and the study of disease (epidemiology). These include measures of disease occurrence, such as risk and incidence, and absolute and relative measures of effect, such as risk difference, relative risk and odds ratio.

**Objectives and learning outcomes**

The objectives for this chapter are to:

- introduce basic measures of disease frequency in population
- discuss the usage of absolute and relative effect measures

After reading this chapter, you should be able to:

- construct frequency tables of disease versus exposure
- use R to calculate various disease and effect measures
- interpret and report the measures of disease and effect appropriately

## 3.1 Key measures of occurrence

### 3.1.1 *Risk*

In everyday language, risk means the possibility of something bad happening. In statistics, risk refers to the probability that a person will experience an event (e.g., a change in health state) within a specified period. For example, we might be interested in the 10-year risk of developing cardiovascular disease, the 5-year risk of dying from cancer, or the risk of becoming seriously ill following an infection. The risk is estimated by dividing the number of events by the number of people *at risk* for the event at the start and followed for the referent time period (Miller and Homan, 1994). Risk varies between zero and one. Terms synonymous with risk include probability, likelihood,[1] and cumulative incidence.

$$\text{risk} = \frac{\text{number of events}}{\text{number of people at risk at start}}$$

*Example: A hypothetical cohort study in diabetes patients*

For example, if we studied 100 people with diabetes for two years, all of whom were at an elevated risk for renal failure at the start of the study (confirmed not to have renal failure already) and found that 10 developed renal failure within the two years, we would estimate the two-year risk of renal failure as $10/100 = 0.1$, or 10%. In practice, being able to follow all the participants in a study is challenging, but statisticians have developed several methods of estimating risk when we cannot follow all participants in a study. The risk and 95% confidence interval can be calculated in R by doing the following:

```
dat <- matrix(c(10,100),ncol=2)
epiR::epi.conf(dat,
               ctype = "inc.risk",
               method = "clopper-pearson")
```

---

[1]Likelihood is also used in mathematical statistics to define a different quantity altogether.

```
##    est       lower      upper
## 1 0.1 0.04900469 0.1762226
```

### 3.1.2  *Rate*

When people in a study are followed for different lengths of time, we tend to calculate rates rather than risk. The rate is the number of events divided by total person-time (the sum of all the follow-up time of people at risk at the start). Examples of rates in medical research include the incidence rate, where the new events are the first occurrence or diagnosis of disease, and the mortality rate, which describes the rate at which deaths occur per unit of time, typically annually. The rate is often denoted by the Greek letter $\lambda$ using the formula

$$\text{rate} = \lambda = \frac{\text{number of events}}{\text{total person-time}}$$

When the event is rare, the rate can be approximated by

$$\lambda \approx \frac{\text{risk up to time } t}{t}$$

*Example: Cohort study in diabetes, continued*

We previously calculated the two-year risk of renal failure in the hypothetical cohort of diabetes patients at 10%. We now calculate the rate of renal failure by dividing the number of events (10) by the total person-time. In a fixed cohort such as this, the person-time contribution for people not developing renal failure is the measurement interval (two years). For the 10 people who developed renal failure, their person-time contribution is the time up to their diagnosis. Table 3.1 shows how the calculations proceed for all people in the cohort. The rate is then $\lambda = 10/184.5 = 0.0542$ per person-year, which is also the *annual* rate. If we multiply the rate by 100, we get 5.42 per 100 person-years. Using the approximation method described earlier, the rate is $0.10/2 = 0.05$, which is close but underestimates the true rate.

**Table 3.1.**  Calculation of person-time in a hypothetical two-year study of incident renal failure in people with diabetes.

| ID | Experienced event (renal failure) | Time of event or last follow-up time | Person-time contribution (in years) |
|----|-----------------------------------|--------------------------------------|-------------------------------------|
| 1 | No | 730 | 2 |
| 2 | Yes | 137 | 0.187 |
| 3 | Yes | 492 | 0.674 |
| ⋮ | ⋮ | ⋮ | ⋮ |
| 100 | No | 730 | 2 |

Total person-time = 184.5

The rate and 95% confidence interval can be calculated in R by doing the following:

```
dat <- matrix(c(10,184.5),ncol=2)

# Incidence rate with 95% confidence interval

epiR::epi.conf(dat,
ctype = "inc.rate",
method = "exact")

##            est        lower        upper
## 1 0.05420054 0.02599127 0.09967673
```

### 3.1.3  *Prevalence*

The prevalence measures how common a condition is in a population. The prevalence is estimated by the number of existing events divided by the total number of people assessed at a particular point in time. In contrast to risk and rates of events, the prevalence relates to a snapshot in time rather than a period of time. It is estimated using the following equation:

$$\text{prevalence} = \frac{\text{number of events}}{\text{number of people}}$$

*Example: Prevalence of new cancer in individuals with Li–Fraumeni syndrome*

In a cohort study of 116 individuals with the Li–Fraumeni syndrome (Mai *et al.*, 2017), baseline cancer screening led to the diagnosis of cancer in eight (6.9%) individuals (two lung, one osteosarcoma, one sarcoma, one astrocytoma, one low-grade glioma, and two pre-invasive breast cancers (DCIS)), with all but one requiring definitive treatment.

```
dat <- matrix(c(8,116),ncol=2)
epiR::epi.conf(dat, ctype = "prevalence",
method = "wilson")*100

##           est     lower     upper
## 1 6.896552 3.535749 13.02067
```

### 3.1.4 *Odds*

The odds of an outcome can be defined as the probability $p$ that the outcome occurs divided by the probability that the outcome does not occur $(1 - p)$. Hence,

$$\text{odds} = \frac{p}{1 - p}$$

If the probability $p$ relates to a risk then the odds are called risk odds. If $p$ relates to a prevalence then they are referred to as prevalence odds.

When the odds are greater than 1.0, the outcome is more likely than not, and when the odds are less than 1.0, the outcome is less likely. Odds of 2.0 mean that the outcome is twice as likely as not. Conversely, if the odds are 0.5, then the outcome is twice as likely *not* to happen. We can convert odds back to risk using the equation

$$\text{risk} = \frac{\text{odds}}{1 + \text{odds}}$$

*Example: Li–Fraumeni syndrome, continued*

Continuing with the previous example. The prevalence odds (95% confidence interval) of new cancer in individuals with the Li–Fraumeni syndrome could be calculated in R as follows:

```
dat <- matrix(c(8,108),ncol=2)
epiR::epi.conf(dat,ctype = "odds")

##          est        lower       upper
## 1 0.07407407 0.02654867 0.1372549
```

### 3.1.5   *Hazard*

In survival analysis, the hazard rate measures the instantaneous risk of an event happening. The events often refer to negative outcomes such as death or progression of disease. The length of time until the event occurs is called the survival time. An average hazard can be calculated by dividing the number of events by the total survival time.

$$\text{average hazard} = \frac{\text{number of events}}{\text{total survival time}}$$

This descriptive measure is seldom used and it is much more common to survival analyses to report hazard ratios rather than summary measures of hazard.

## 3.2   Measures of effect

This section covers some common absolute and relative measures of effect. Some controversy surrounds whether risk information should be presented in relative or absolute terms. This is because relative measures of risk, although appealing because they summarise two numbers into one, obscure the absolute risk, and tend to exaggerate the benefits of treatments and interventions (Noordzij *et al.*, 2017). On the other hand, it has been argued that only presenting absolute risks and risk differences could incorrectly lead to a treatment or intervention being considered unimportant. We recommend you present both absolute and relative measures when communicating risk.

### 3.2.1 *Risk difference or attributable risk*

The attributable risk provides a measure of excess risk in absolute terms. It is simply the difference in risk between the two groups. For example, if we measure the risk of some outcome in an exposed group and the risk of the same outcome in an unexposed group, the risk difference is

$$\text{risk difference} = \text{risk(exposed)} - \text{risk(unexposed)}$$

*Example: Exemestane for breast cancer prevention*

In a trial of exemestane for breast cancer prevention in post-menopausal women, the risk of invasive breast cancer in the treatment (exemestane) group was $11/2285 = 0.0048$ and $32/2275 = 0.014$ in the placebo group (Goss *et al.*, 2011). The risk difference is therefore $0.0048 - 0.014 = -0.0092$.

### 3.2.2 *Population attributable fraction*

The population attributable fraction (PAF) or attributable fraction (AF) is the proportion of disease in a population that can be attributed to a risk factor or exposure. It can be found by determining how many more cases occur in a group exposed to some risk as a fraction of the total number of cases in a population. Suppose we wanted to calculate the attributable fraction of ischaemic heart disease in men who smoked 15–24 cigarettes per day. We would need to know how many men did or did not smoke, and how many cases of ischaemic heart disease occurred in each group. Suppose there are 1000 smokers and 10000 non-smokers in a population, and 450 cases of ischaemic heart disease in non-smokers and 100 in the smokers. It is reasonable to suppose that in the absence of any increased risk from smoking, the smokers would have the same underlying rate of disease as the non-smokers. Using this logic, we can say that we would expect $1000 \times 450/10000 = 45$ cases of ischaemic heart disease in the men who smoke. As we have observed 100 cases of ischaemic heart disease in the men who smoke then we could say that there were

$100 - 45 = 55$ more cases than we would have expected. The difference can be attributed to the smoking if we are confident that the two groups are comparable in their risk of ischaemic heart disease in every other sense. The attributable fraction is then this number divided by the total number of cases of ischaemic heart disease;

$$\text{AF} = \frac{100 - 45}{100 + 450} = 10\%$$

The fraction of ischaemic heart disease attributed to smoking in this setting is therefore 10%.

### 3.2.3   *Number needed to treat/harm*

The number needed to treat (NNT) is a measure that indicates how many patients on average need to be treated in order to benefit one patient

$$\text{NNT} = \frac{1}{|\text{risk difference}|}$$

*Example: Exemestane for for breast cancer prevention, continued*

The NNT for exemestane is, therefore, $1/0.0092 = 109$. We could interpret this as, on average, for every 109 women treated with this drug, we would expect one fewer invasive breast cancer. As the NNT is based on a risk, it is also wise to quote the time period to which it refers; here, in this example, the median follow-up is 35 months. Above all others, the NNT statistic divides opinion and has attracted its fair share of critics (see, for example, Hutton (2000)). Some make a convincing case for it as a means of communication (see, for example, Altman (1998)). We should caution that the NNT should not be taken literally; it does not mean you *need* to treat 109 patients to prevent one invasive breast cancer, but instead that in treating 109 patients, we would expect to avoid one invasive breast cancer.

When dealing with a bad outcome, NNT becomes 'the number needed to treat for harm', or NNTH.

### 3.2.4  *Risk ratio*

Relative measures of effect involve dividing one effect measure by another. The resulting ratio, therefore, provides a measure of the relative difference between two effect measures. The relative risk, or risk ratio, is the ratio of two risk estimates. The risk ratio could be used to compare the risk of a bad outcome without treatment to the risk of a bad outcome under treatment. A risk ratio of less than one would indicate that the treatment group had a lower risk of a bad outcome, and a number greater than one would suggest that the risk is higher under treatment.

*Example: A fictional trial of a new drug*

Suppose a trial is carried out to see if a new drug can reduce the risk of heart attack or stroke in people who already have heart disease. The risk of dying from a heart attack or stroke was reported to be 4 per 100 in the usual care group and 3 per 100 in the treatment group. The risk ratio is, therefore

$$\text{risk ratio} = \frac{3/100}{4/100} = 0.75$$

The relative risk reduction could be calculated as follows:

$$\left(\frac{4-3}{4}\right) \times 100 = 25\%$$

### 3.2.5  *Odds ratio*

The ratio of two odds is called the odds ratio (OR). The disease odds ratio is defined as

$$\text{disease OR} = \frac{\text{odds of disease in exposed}}{\text{odds of disease in unexposed}}$$

An odds ratio OR > 1 would mean the disease is more common in the exposed group than in the unexposed group. An OR < 1 would mean the disease is less likely to occur in the exposed group than in the unexposed group. An OR = 1 means that the disease is equally likely in the exposed as it is in the unexposed.

*Example: Fictional trial, continued*

The odds of dying from a heart attack or stroke is 3/97 under treatment and 4/96 under usual care. The odds ratio is, therefore,

$$OR = (3/97)/(4/96) = 0.742$$

The odds of dying from a heart attack or stroke under treatment is 74% of the odds of dying from a heart attack or stroke under usual care. This means that the treatment decreases the odds of dying by 26% as compared to under usual care. Conversely, the odds ratio of not dying from a heart attack or stroke is $1/0.742 = 1.347$. That is, the treatment increases the odds of not dying by 35% as compared to usual care. The two statements are equivalent and have the same conclusions.

The OR of dying (0.742) is very close to the risk ratio (0.75). This is not a coincidence. Typically, when the risk is low ($<10\%$) the odds ratio is similar to the risk ratio.

### 3.2.6 Rate ratio

The ratio of two rates is called a relative rate or rate ratio. They provide a relative measure of the difference in rates between the two groups. For a rare outcome,

$$\text{risk} \approx \text{odds} \approx \text{rate} \times \text{time}$$

and, therefore, it is also true that when the outcome is rare,

$$\text{risk ratio} \approx \text{odds ratio} \approx \text{rate ratio}$$

For more common outcomes, the three measures will be different (Kirkwood and Sterne, 2010).

### 3.2.7 Hazard ratio

The hazard ratio is a measure of effect used almost exclusively in survival or time-to-event analyses. Although different from an OR, it is interpreted similarly. A hazard ratio of 1 corresponds to an equal hazard and no effect. A hazard ratio greater than 1 would mean the comparator group has a higher hazard, whereas less than 1 would mean a lower hazard than the reference group. For example, a hazard ratio of 0.5 would imply that the hazard in the comparator group is half that of the reference group. In the special case where all failure times are observed, a *crude* hazard ratio is given, dividing the average hazard in the comparator group by the average hazard in the reference group. In nearly all practical examples, the failure times will not be known for all participants, and the hazard ratio will need to be estimated using methods that take missing failure times into account.

### 3.2.8    *Choosing between effect measures*

In longitudinal studies in which data on times to event are recorded, the rate ratios (including hazard ratios) tend to be the preferred effect measure, particularly if follow-up is incomplete or individuals enter cohorts at different points in time and are followed for differing lengths of time (i.e., dynamic cohorts). Both risk and odds ratios can be estimated from longitudinal studies with complete follow-up (Kirkwood and Sterne, 2010). In cross-sectional studies, odds ratios and estimates of prevalence are common. The only appropriate measure of effect in a case-control study is the OR.

### 3.2.9    *Effect measure or measure of association*

While the terms 'effect measure' and 'measures of association' are often used interchangeably, some authors distinguish the two terms (Greenland and Lash, 2008). The term 'effect measure' is reserved for direct estimates of effect from randomised trials and causal inference studies, while 'measures of association' is used for observational comparisons. For example, comparing the difference in the rates of dental caries in children before and after the introduction of fluoridation would be a measure of association. In contrast, a rate difference estimated from a randomised trial of fluoridation would be considered an effect measure.

### 3.3    Calculating measures of effect in R

We finish this chapter by showing how to calculate ORs, relative risks, and rate ratios in R. In Chapter 5, we go into more detail and

**Table 3.2.** A generic two-way table for odds and risk calculation.

|                    | Event   | Non-event | Total   |
|--------------------|---------|-----------|---------|
| Comparator group   | $a$     | $b$       | $a + b$ |
| Reference group    | $c$     | $d$       | $c + d$ |
| Total              | $a + c$ | $b + d$   | $N$     |

show functions that can carry out tests and hypotheses and calculate confidence intervals for these measures. For now, we focus solely on descriptive measures.

### 3.3.1 *Two-way tables*

To calculate risk and odds ratios, we require two independent groups, with the number of events that occurred and did not occur for both groups. The comparator group could represent people exposed to some agent or treatment in a trial, and the reference group could consist of people not exposed or given a placebo or standard care. This arrangement has four cells ($a, b, c,$ and $d$) as per Table 3.2.

For rate ratios the non-event column is replaced with total person-time.

### 3.3.2 *Calculation*

A two-way table can be entered into R using either the `matrix()` function or by binding (by column or row) two vectors. Naming the rows and columns, using the `dimnames()` function is optional but useful for checking you have entered the data correctly.

```
# some arbitrary numbers
a <- 50
b <- 113
c <- 34
d <- 69
tab <- matrix(c(a,c,b,d), 2, 2)
dimnames(tab) <- list(
Group = c("Comparator","Reference"),
"Outcome" = c("Event", "Non-event")
)
```

```
tab
```

```
##              Outcome
## Group        Event Non-event
##    Comparator   50      113
##    Reference    34       69
```

The effect measure calculation proceeds as follows using the `epi.2by2()` function from the `epiR` package;

```
r <- epiR::epi.2by2(tab,
method = "cohort.count")

# risk ratio/odds ratio/AF statistics
r$massoc.summary

# All metrics including NNT.
r$massoc.detail
```

## 3.4   Problems and exercises

(1) Of 934 people who were known to be free of a particular disease at the start of a study, 39 developed the disease within two years. Assuming the status of all 934 were known at the end of the study, estimate the cumulative incidence and 95% confidence interval for these data.

(2) Investigators of a study enrolled 2100 children and followed them for three years to determine the incidence rate of type 1 diabetes mellitus (T1DM). After one year, none had a new diagnosis of T1DM, but 100 children had been lost to follow-up. After two years, one had a new diagnosis of T1DM, and another 50 had been lost to follow-up. In the final year, there was one more new diagnosis of T1DM, and 250 had been lost to follow-up. Calculate the annual incidence rate (per 100000) and 95% confidence interval of T1DM. Assume that the cases and those lost to follow-up contribute half-year follow-up (i.e., the actuarial method).

(3) The `Remission` dataset from the `R4HCR` package has data on the duration of remission for acute leukaemia patients on active

treatment or placebo. Estimate the average hazard of 'relapse' in the placebo group.

(4) Suppose a population was studied to establish the number of people with cataracts. In this study, 2352 were examined, and cataracts were reported in 278 individuals (either or both eyes). Estimate the prevalence and 95% Wilson score confidence interval of cataracts in this population.

(5) Suppose the test used in the previous study was imperfect and tended to miss cataracts when they were present 90% of the time and incorrectly say people had cataracts when they didn't 5% of the time. Compute the true prevalence of cataracts. (*Hint*: Use the `epi.prev` function from the `epiR` package to do this.)

(6) The Coronary Drug Project was a randomised, double-blind trial conducted to assess the effects of five cholesterol drugs on mortality in men. The five-year mortality for one drug, clofibrate, compared to the placebo, is shown in Table 3.3.

**Table 3.3.** Five-year mortality results from the Coronary Drug randomised control trial.

|  | Died | Total ($n$) |
| --- | --- | --- |
| Clofibrate | 194 | 1065 |
| Placebo | 521 | 2695 |
| Total | 715 | 3760 |

(a) Use hand calculation (i.e., not using R packages) to estimate risks and odds of death for each of the two groups, and express the results as fractions.

(b) Estimate the relative risk, risk difference, and odds ratio, comparing the clofibrate group with the placebo group. Perform hand calculations. Write a sentence to interpret each of the measures.

(c) Calculate by hand the attributable proportion or prevention proportions (depending on which is more appropriate) and interpret the result.

(7) We stated that OR(disease) = 1/OR(healthy), using the example in Section 3.2.4, show that this holds for an odds ratio but this is not true for the risk ratio.

(8) In a trial of two treatments to reduce breast cancer risk, there were 163 cases of invasive breast cancer in the women assigned to tamoxifen and 168 cases in those assigned to raloxifene (Vogel *et al.*, 2006), if the total follow-up in the two groups was 37895 and 38105 person-years respectively, what are the rates per 1000 in each group and the rate ratio for raloxifene versus tamoxifen.

(9) In a study of a weight loss drug (semaglutide) in overweight or obese adults, a total of 1961 participants were randomly assigned to receive semaglutide ($N = 1306$) or placebo ($N = 655$).

    (a) Among the participants for whom data were available at the week 68 visit (1212 participants in the semaglutide group and 577 in the placebo group), 612 on semaglutide and 28 on placebo achieved a weight loss of 15%. Calculate the odds ratio corresponding to weight loss on semaglutide versus placebo.

    (b) The same publication reported that serious adverse events were reported in 128 (9.8%) and 42 (6.4%) serious adverse events were reported in semaglutide and placebo arms respectively. Use these data to calculate the number needed to 'treat for harm' for semaglutide.

# Chapter 4

# Displaying data

One of the strengths of R is its ability to produce high-quality graphics and charts, from simple *high-level* plots that let you quickly and easily display your data to sophisticated bespoke graphics. In this chapter, we first demonstrate the five key high-level plots used in healthcare research (bar chart, box plot, histogram, scatter, and Q–Q plot) and how to modify them. We finish this chapter by showing you the *low-level* or modular approach to creating graphs using only base R functions.

**Objectives and learning outcomes**

The objectives for this chapter are to:

- describe the five most used plotting functions in base R
- show how to customise basic plot types
- build a plot from first principles using a modular approach

After reading this chapter, you should be able to:

- use R to create high-quality graphical summaries of data
- construct plots using base R functions in a modular approach
- save and export graphs in multiple formats, including .png, .jpeg, and .pdf

## 4.1  Bar chart

### 4.1.1  *Overview*

A bar chart displays data which have been or *can be* classified into nominal or ordinal categories. Rectangular bars of equal width are drawn (c.f. to histogram) for each category, with the heights equal to the category's frequency. The core R function to draw a bar chart is `barplot()`.

### 4.1.2  *Data requirements*

The type of bar chart R draws depends on the object's class supplied to its main argument `height`. Objects can be either a vector, array or matrix. If a vector is supplied, R will draw a sequence of bars with heights corresponding to the values in the vector. If a matrix or array is given, a stacked bar chart or side-by-side bar chart can be produced – using the `beside` argument. For bar plots stratified by a factor or factors, the user can specify a formula-style argument:

```
# option 1
# a vector heights (h) and a categorical variable x
# x is used to label the bars
barplot(h ~ x, data = dt)


# option 2
# a vector of heights, and 2 categorical
# variables x1 and x2
barplot(h ~ x1 + x2, data = dt)


# option 3
# two frequencies (y1 and y2) and
# one categorical variable x
barplot(cbind(y1, y2) ~ x, data = dt)
```

Option 1 will draw bars of height $h$ and label the bars with values in $x$. Option 2 will cross-tabulate $x1$ and $x2$ with $x1$ nested within $x2$, meaning that the categories of $x1$ will be either stacked or placed side by side for each level of $x2$. Option 3 will stack or place side by side two frequencies for each category of $x$.

### 4.1.3   Modifications

#### 4.1.3.1   Positioning of bars

If a matrix or array is supplied to the **height** argument, the data in each column of the matrix or array can displayed as stacked bars, or juxtaposed bars. Specify **beside = F** for stacked and **beside = T** for juxtaposed. If the data are proportions then it can be useful to stack bars rather than juxtapose.

#### 4.1.3.2   Adjusting and labelling bars

R will default to adding the attribute of the height vector or column names (if a matrix is supplied) below each bar or group of bars. This can be overwritten by providing a vector of names to the **names.arg** argument. More space (as a fraction of the average bar width) can be added between the bars using the **barplot(..., space = X)** argument. Values greater than 1 will add space, whereas values less than 1 will move the bars closer together. The **width** argument does not change the width of the bar visually but instead changes the scale of the $x$ values and the midpoints of the bars. The midpoints can be accessed by saving the bar chart as an object (see the following code) and then calling it. The values returned are the midpoints; we can use this to label and position the legend, etc.

```
heights <- c(1,2,3,4,5)
bp1 <- barplot(heights,width = 1,plot=F)
bp2 <- barplot(heights,width = 2,plot=F)
data.frame('width of 1' = bp1,'width of 2' = bp2)

##    width.of.1 width.of.2
## 1        0.7        1.4
## 2        1.9        3.8
## 3        3.1        6.2
## 4        4.3        8.6
## 5        5.5       11.0
```

Labelling the bars with frequencies can be done using this trick. First, save the plot as an R object, and then use the `text()` command to add labels. Setting the $y$-axis coordinate to 0 means the labels will be set at the bottom of the bars. The `labels` should be a character string vector of the same length as the number of bars.

```
bp1 <- barplot(heights)
text(x = bp1, y = 0, labels = mylabels)
```

### 4.1.3.3   *Adjusting axes*

The limits of the $x$ and $y$ axes can be controlled using the `xlim = c(min, max)` and `ylim = c(min, max)` arguments. Labels for the $x$-axis are controlled using the `ylab = ""` and `xlab = ""` options. Axes can be switched off using the `xaxt = "n"` or `yaxt = "n"` or `axes=F` options. Use the option `las = 2` to rotate the $x$ label text by 90 degrees. The default is `las = 1`, which means the labels are horizontal.

### 4.1.3.4   *Shading and colour*

The bars of the plot can be coloured in using the `col` argument. The 'RColorBrewer package' has a variety of sequential and diverging colour palettes, which make this easier.

```
library(RColorBrewer)
cols <- brewer.pal(n = 5,name = "Spectral")
barplot(Scot,...,col = cols,...)
```

The option, `border` can be used to colour the border of the bars (or use `border = NA` to omit borders). Use the `density` argument to control the density of shading lines (in lines per inch) and the `angle` argument to modify the angle (in degrees) of the slope of shading lines.

### 4.1.3.5   *Scaling*

Scaling is controlled using the `cex` arguments. Use `cex.names` to change the size of the bar labels and `cex.axis` to adjust the size of the value of the frequency axis. Values less than one will reduce the size, while values greater than one will increase the size. Scaling of the legend text can be controlled within the **args.legend** argument.

### 4.1.3.6 *Legends*

If more than one set of frequencies is presented, it makes sense to provide a legend to help identify which colour is represented. Use the **legend.text** argument for this. For positioning and scaling, use **args.legend**, e.g.,

```
# M is matrix containing two frequencies.
barplot(M,
...,
legend.text = c("",""),
args.legend = c(x = 10, y = 90, cex = 0.9, ncol = 2,...)
)
```

A large number of parameters can be modified within the **arg.legend** argument; for a complete list, see the help page for **legend**.

### 4.1.4 *Examples*

#### 4.1.4.1 *Example 1: Simple bar chart*

The **Vaccinated** dataset has the number of people per hundred vaccinated against COVID-19 per the week ending 12 November 2021 for European countries with a population greater than 10 million. The simple plot is obtained as follows (Figure 4.1):

```
data(Vaccinated, package = "R4HCR")
heights <- Vaccinated$vaccinated
names <- Vaccinated$country
bp <- barplot(height = heights,
col = "white",
ylim=c(0,100),
names.arg = names,
```

```
cex.names = 0.9,
las = 2,
ylab = "People vaccinated per 100")

# using round() to show integers on plot
labels <- round(Vaccinated$vaccinated,0)

text(x = bp, y = labels-2, labels = labels,
cex = 0.9, pos = 3)
```

### 4.1.4.2   *Example 2: More than one frequency per category*

To show more than one set of frequencies per category, we must create a matrix or array: two vectors stacked or bound together. The shape of the matrix or array will determine how the data are plotted. We create a matrix with two columns: one for vaccination rates and the other for 'fully' vaccinated rates per country. In R, we can do this as follows (Figure 4.2):

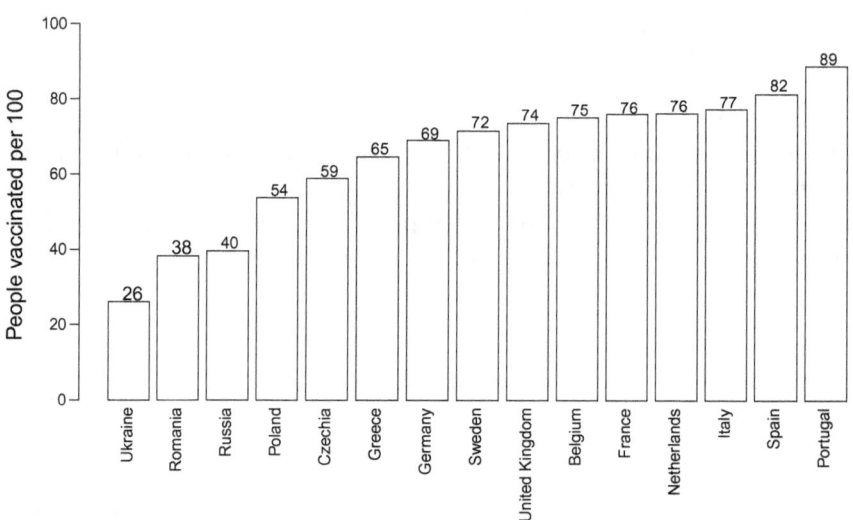

**Fig. 4.1.**   A bar chart of vaccination rates across European countries.

```
r1 <- Vaccinated$vaccinated # frequency 1
r2 <- Vaccinated$fully_vaccinated  # frequency 2

# rbind() binds or stacks the two vectors
Mat <- rbind(r1,r2)

# 2 rows and 15 columns
dim(Mat)

# as an alternative to supplying a names argument
# we add the location (country) names as column names
# to our array.
colnames(Mat) <- Vaccinated$country

# note the positioning of the legend in arg.legend()
barplot(height = Mat,
beside = T,
cex.names = 0.7,
las = 2,
ylab = "People vaccinated per 100",
legend.text = c("Vaccinated","Fully vaccinated"),
args.legend = c(x = 16, y = 90, cex = 0.9))
```

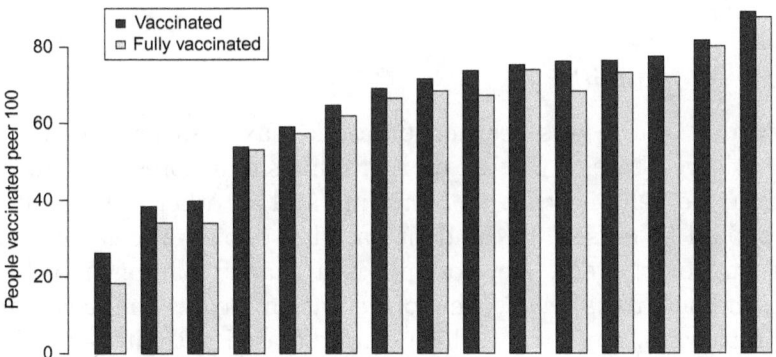

**Fig. 4.2.** A side-by-side bar chart; vaccinated versus fully vaccinated rates in 15 European countries.

### 4.1.4.3  *Example 3: A stacked bar chart*

An alternative way to present category data with more than one
set of frequencies is by stacking the bars rather than placing them
side by side. This can help draw out a trend if, for example, the $x$-
axis represents time. We illustrate this using the Scotland mortality
data Scot, which has the number of people death registrations per
week for the first 42 weeks of 2021, broken down by cause of death.
By stacking the bars, the trends can be seen more easily and more
efficiently with space (Figure 4.3).

```
data(Scotland, package="R4HCR")

# it has this many rows and columns
dim(Scotland)

# Find a colour palette
colr <- RColorBrewer::brewer.pal(5, "Set3")

barplot(Scotland,
col = colr,
legend.text = c("Cancer","Dementia/Alzheimers",
"Circulatory/Respiratory","Covid-19","Other"),
beside = F,
cex.names = 0.8,
args.legend = c(ncol = 3, cex = 0.75, x = 45))
```

### 4.1.5  *Comments*

Edward R. Tufte was keen on data-ink maximisation and believed
that a large share of the ink on a graphic should present data information. He believed that *non-data* ink and all other redundant data
ink should be erased. Redundant data-ink depicts the same number
over and over again. An example is a shaded bar on a bar chart
with the heights labelled. This presentation locates the height in six
separate ways, any five of which can be erased without redundancy:

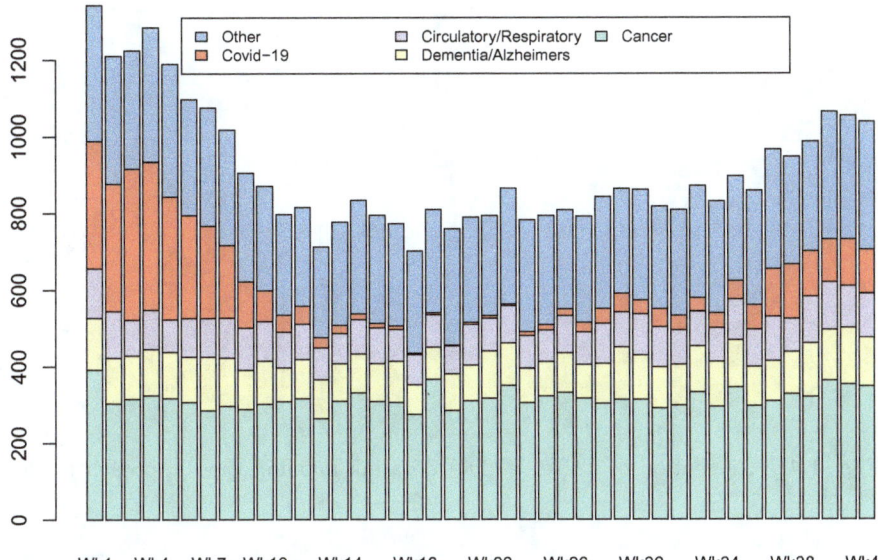

**Fig. 4.3.** Example of a stacked barchart: Mortality in the first 42 weeks of 2021 by causes of death.

(1) the height of the left line, (2) the height of the shading, (3) the height of the right line, (4) the position of the top horizontal line, and (5) the position of number at the bar's top and the number itself (Tufte, 2001). He was also critical of chart junk and probably would have been critical of the hatching in Figure 4.3. An example of this style applied to a bar chart is recreated here (Figure 4.4). What is your opinion of Tufte's version – is it comprehensible?

```
y <- c(9,12,6,7,3,18,14,9,6,11,5,10)
barplot(y,col = "gray",yaxt="n",
        border = "white",space = 1.5)
abline(h = c(5,10,15), col = "white")
abline(h=0,col = "gray")
mtext(text = paste(c(5,10,15),"%"),
side = 2,line = 1,at = c(5,10,15),las = 2)
```

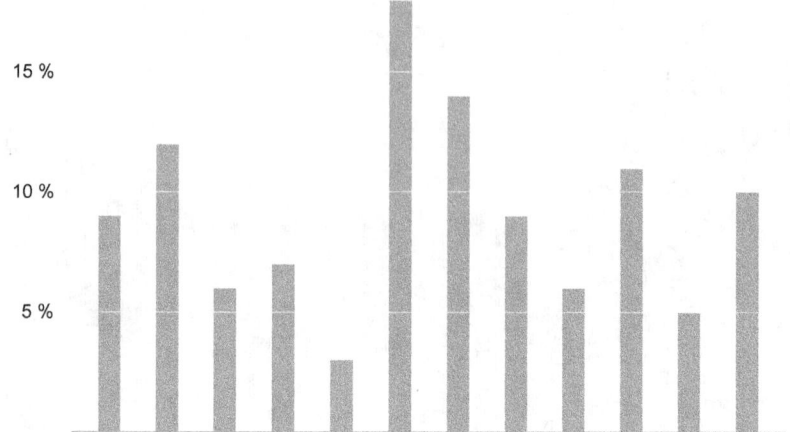

**Fig. 4.4.** Recreation of Tufte's (2001) data-ink maximisation approach to the bar chart.

## 4.2 Histogram

### 4.2.1 *Overview*

A histogram is a helpful way to visualise data distribution. It can help locate outliers or errant values, check symmetry, and help determine if the distribution has multiple modes. Central tendency and spread or *variability* are also readily seen in the histogram. The base R function for a histogram `hist(x, ...)` is highly flexible, with many options to enhance the base plot.

### 4.2.2 *Data requirements*

The first argument to the `hist()` function is `x`, a vector of values for which the histogram is desired. This can be a numeric vector or a matrix – a matrix will be treated as a vector.

The default is the intervals for the histogram cells to be right-closed (left-open) (`right = T`). A value of 1, with breaks of `breaks = c(0,1,2)`, will fall within the 0-1 bin rather than the 1-2 bin. If `right=F` is selected, then a value of 1 will fall within the 1-2 bin.

```
x <- 1
```

```
# the default
h <- hist(x, breaks=c(0,1,2),right=T,plot=F)
h$counts
```

```
## [1] 1 0
```

```
j <- hist(x, breaks=c(0,1,2),right=F,plot=F)
j$counts
```

```
## [1] 0 1
```

The option `include.lowest = T` is self-explanatory. If the lowest value in the data coincides with the lowest break value, it will be included in the first bar rather than being excluded and forcing an error.

### 4.2.3 *Modifications*

4.2.3.1 *Choice of binwidth or breaks*

According to the R help page, this can be one of the following:

- a vector giving the breakpoints between histogram cells
- a function to compute the vector of breakpoints
- a single number giving the number of cells for the histogram
- a character string naming an algorithm to compute the number of cells
- a function to compute the number of cells.

```
# A vector of breakpoints
hist(x, breaks = seq(0,200,20))
```

```
# A function for breakpoints
hist(x, breaks = function(x) seq(min(x),max(x),20))
```

```
# A single number no of cells
# a suggestion only; as the breakpoints will be set
```

```
# to pretty values - see comments.
hist(x, breaks = 12)

# String stating algorithm, defaults to Sturges
hist(x, breaks = "FD")

# function for number of cells,
# x vector is supplied to it as the only argument
hist(x, breaks = function(x) sqrt(length(x)))
```

### 4.2.3.2　Adjusting the y and x axes

The default is for the $y$-axis to be the frequency or counts of observations within each bin or class interval. The alternative is to use the probability density scale and obtain a 'true' histogram (a *true* histogram has a density area equal to 1). The MASS library has a function called truehist() which defaults to this, but to obtain a histogram with the $y$-axis on the density scale with the hist() function, use freq = F or probability = T. Y-axis limits are controlled using the ylim argument. The limits of the $x$-axis can be controlled using the xlim argument. Labels for the axes are controlled using the xlab and ylab options. Axes can be switched off using the axes = F option.

### 4.2.3.3　Shading and colour

The colours of the bars are selected using the col argument, whereas the borders of the bars are set using the border argument. Shading lines can be added using the density argument, with large positive values producing more shading lines; the angle of these lines can be adjusted using the angle option (degrees counter-clockwise).

### 4.2.3.4　Legends

Legends can be added to most, if not all, base R plots using the legend() function in a separate line after executing the initial plot command, e.g.,

```
hist(x,...)
legend(x =, y =, legend="blah")
```

This function gives fine control over the positioning and style of the legend, but the user will need to supply the text, line types, and colours. A character string or $x$–$y$ coordinates can specify the legend's position. The character string can be one of 'bottomright', 'bottom', 'bottomleft', 'left', 'topleft', 'top', 'topright', 'right', or 'center'. Coordinates are on the native scale and not relative (0–1 range). A helpful trick to quickly locate the position of your legend is to run the plot command and then use the `locator()` function, e.g.,

```
locator()
```

which will bring up a hatch on the plot window. With your mouse, click on the desired location(s) and then press escape; you should find the $x$ and $y$ coordinates printed in the console.

The **legend** argument (the second argument within the **legend()** function) refers to a character or expression vector of length $\geq 1$; this is what will be used as labels for the lines or points you want to identify. These two arguments are the minimum required for the legend to be added to the plot, but further modifications are possible.

```
# first plot something, then

legend("topleft",
legend = c("series 1","series 2"),
col = 1:2, # colours
lty = 1:2,  # line type
pch = 16:17, # can have points and lines
inset = 0.05, # move box inside 0.05 units
bty = "n", # don't have a surrounding box
title = "Legend title", # Add a title to the legend box
ncol = 1,  # have 1 or more columns
)
```

### 4.2.3.5 *Further modifications*

The `labels=T` argument adds labels above the bars, either the counts/frequencies or the density values if the `freq = F` option is selected. A title can be added using the `main` option. Use `main = NULL` to suppress the title.

## 4.2.4 *Examples*

### 4.2.4.1 *Example 1: Simple histogram*

The default is for the $y$-axis to be the frequency or counts of observations within each bin or class interval. We demonstrate this using the SCAN dataset, which has blood test results taken on people presenting to primary care with vague symptoms that could be cancer. For this example, we look at the haemoglobin test results. Because there are a few outliers, the default Sturges algorithm leads to class intervals of 20, which is quite wide. We can request smaller class intervals using the $\sqrt{n}$ rule by invoking the `nclass` argument (Figure 4.5).

```
data(SCAN, package="R4HCR")

hist(SCAN$haemoglobin,
nclass = sqrt(nrow(SCAN)),
main = NULL,
xlab = "Haemoglobin (g/L)")
```

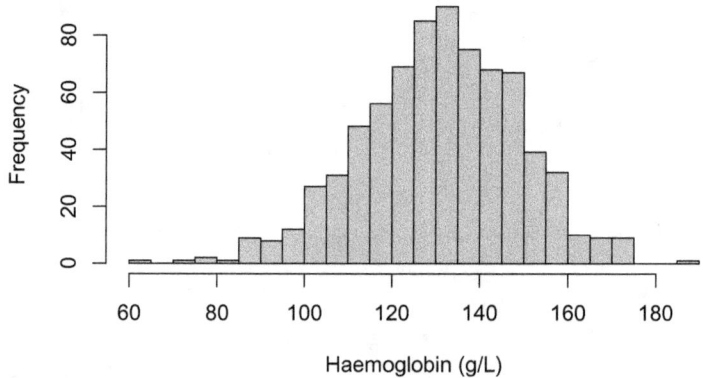

**Fig. 4.5.** Histogram of the haemoglobin values from the SCAN dataset.

Opting for `freq = F` means the *y*-axis is scaled as a density. The total area of all the bars in the plot now sums to 1. The height of each bar is determined by the number of observations within a bin multiplied by its width, and then divided by the total number of observations.

### 4.2.4.2  *Example 2: Histogram with overlaid normal density*

It can sometimes be helpful to add a curve from a theoretical probability distribution to the histogram. Typically, this theoretical distribution will be normal, but other probability distributions can also be used. To add a density curve to a histogram in R, first draw a histogram making sure to set freq = F, and then use **curve()** and the density function corresponding to the probability distribution you wish to superimpose over the data. For the haemoglobin data, we would do

```
hist(x, probability = T, nclass = sqrt(length(x)),
main = NULL, xlab = NULL)

# Huber M-estimator of location -
hub <- MASS::huber(x)

# overlay the Normal density.
curve(dnorm(x, hub$mu, hub$s),
from = min(x), to = max(x), add = T)
```

Here (Figure 4.6), we use the Huber M-estimator (**huber()**) of the mean and sample standard deviation, as the usual estimator (the mean in particular) is strongly influenced by the outlying low haemoglobin values in this example.

### 4.2.4.3  *Example 3: Histograms with small data*

For small datasets, the appearance of the histogram can change substantially according to the number and/or width of the bins (Montgomery, 2001). An alternative method is to use a stem-and-leaf plot using the **stem()** function. These not only show the distribution but also give more detail. Like a histogram, the data can be divided into bins, but each data value is split into a 'stem', which is often the first digit, and a 'leaf', which in R is a digit that identifies and

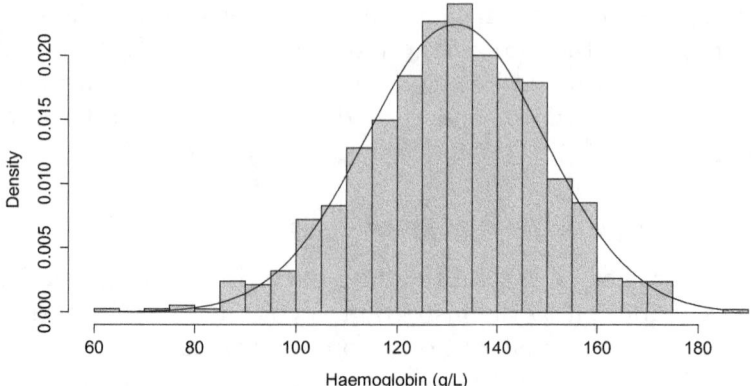

**Fig. 4.6.**   Histogram of haemoglobin data with normal density overlaid.

tallies individual values within each bin. The 'stem' values are listed down, while the 'leaf' values extend right from the stems.

```
# A stem diagram of some random data
y <- c(3,1.21,7,2,2,1.1,5)
stem(y)

##
##    The decimal point is at the |
##
##    0 | 12
##    2 | 000
##    4 | 0
##    6 | 0
```

In this example, the values of 1.21 and 1.1 are represented in the 0 bin, as they fall between 0 and 2 and are identified by the first digit after the decimal place. The stem() function will change the position of the bar (relative to the decimal point) to accommodate large numbers.

### 4.2.5   *Comments*

Histograms can be sensitive to the choice of the number and width of the bins. R defaults to the 'Sturges' algorithm, which implicitly bases bin sizes on the range of the data. Hence, outliers may affect the range and inflate the bin width at the centre of the distribution

(Venables and Ripley, 2002). Other options are 'Scott' and 'FD' (for Freedman–Diaconis). Montgomery (2001) suggests 'that between 5 and 20 bins is satisfactory in most cases and that the number of bins should increase with $n$. Choosing the number of bins approximately equal to the square root of the number of observations often works well in practice'. Unequal bin width is to be avoided as it can create a false impression of data distribution. Sometimes, the frequencies in each bin are divided by the total number of observations, and then the vertical scale of the histogram represents relative frequencies. Rectangles are drawn over each bin, and the height of each rectangle is proportional to the frequency (or the relative frequency).

## 4.3   Box plot

### 4.3.1   *Overview*

Another common way to display data is a box-and-whisker plot (or box plot). In base R, a box plot can be drawn using the function `boxplot()`. A box plot is a useful way to visualise the location, spread and shape of the distribution of a set of data.

The thick line inside the box is the sample median, and the bottom and the top of the box are the upper and lower hinge values (Figure 4.7). The hinges are identical to the lower (Q1) and

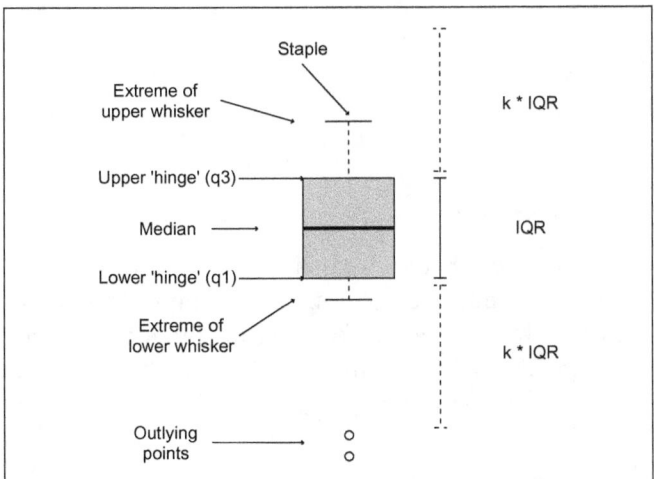

**Fig. 4.7.**  The constituent parts of the box plot.

upper (Q3) quartiles of the data when there is an odd number of
data points but not when there is an even number of data points.
For the most part, the difference is not important. The whiskers
extend out according to the value $k$ or its range. If $k = 0$, the
lower and higher whiskers extend to the lowest or highest value
in the data, respectively. For positive $k$, the whiskers extend out
only as far as the lowest value of $x$ that is greater than $Q1 - k \times$
inter-quartile range (IQR) for the lower whisker and the highest value of $x$ that is less than $Q3 + k \times IQR$ for the highest
whisker.

```
# for data x
k <- 2 # the range variable
bxs <- fivenum(x) # gives the upper and lower hinges.

upper_hinge <- bxs[4]
lower_hinge <- bxs[2]
iqr <- upper_hinge - lower_hinge
lwext <- lower_hinge - k*iqr
uwext <- upper_hinge + k*iqr

# these are how far the whiskers will extend

# lower whisker
min(x[x > lwext])

# upper whisker
max(x[x < uwext])
```

### 4.3.2   *Data requirements*

A box plot is suitable for interval scale data or ordinal scale data. As
per the `hist()` and `barplot()` functions, the data can be supplied
in the form of a single vector. Formula arguments can be made for
box plots of $y$ stratified by a categorical factor $f$. Note that missing
values are ignored in `boxplot()`.

```
# Assuming that x, f1 and f2 are contained
# in a data frame 'dt'

# option 1  - boxplot of single continous variable x
boxplot(x, data = dt)

# option 2a single continuous variable stratified
# by categorical variable f
boxplot(x ~ f1, data = dt)

# option 2b single continuous variable stratified by
# two categorical variables f1 and f2
boxplot(x ~ f1 + f2, data = dt)
```

### 4.3.3  Modifications

#### 4.3.3.1  Orientation

The default orientation is for the boxes to be presented vertically, but use the `horizontal = FALSE` option to have the boxes laid horizontally.

#### 4.3.3.2  Scaling and annotating the boxes

To reduce the width of the boxes, use the `boxwex` argument, and to adjust the width of the staple (the line drawn at the end of the whisker), use `staplewex`. Line types can differ for the whisker, the box, and the median. Use `whisklty` for whisker line types and `lty` for changing the box and median line type.

#### 4.3.3.3  Adjusting the axes

Axis labels and limits are as in Sections 4.1.3.3 and 4.2.3.2: use `xlim`, `ylim`, `xlab`, and `ylab`.

#### 4.3.3.4  Shading and colour

A wide range of options to adjust the parts of the box plot are available in the `boxplot()` function. In general, add `wex` for scaling, `lwd`

**Table 4.1.** Scaling, line type and width, point expansion, and colour options available in `boxplot()`.

| Component | Box | Median | Whisker |
|---|---|---|---|
| Scale factor | boxwex | - | - |
| Line width | boxlwd | medlwd | whisklwd |
| Line type | boxlty | medlty | whisklty |
| Point character | - | medpch | - |
| Point expansion | - | medcex | - |
| Colour | boxcol | medcol | whiskcol |
| Background colour | boxfill | medbg | - |

| Component | Staple | Outlier |
|---|---|---|
| Scale factor | staplewex | outwex |
| Line width | staplelwd | outlwd |
| Line type | staplelty | outlty |
| Point character | - | outpch |
| Point expansion | - | outcex |
| Colour | staplecol | outcol |
| Background colour | - | outbg |

for line width, `lty` for line type, `cex` for point expansion, and `col` and `bg` for colour (see Table 4.1).

#### 4.3.3.5  *Legends*

See Section 4.2.3.4.

### 4.3.4  *Examples*

#### 4.3.4.1  *Example 1: Simple box plot*

Alanine Transaminase (ALT) is an enzyme primarily found in the liver and is a measure of liver cell damage. Here, we first draw box plot of the ALT test results from the SCAN dataset. A first attempt showed a long tail of points extending to the right, suggesting that a log transformation might be beneficial. We can use the `log` option to

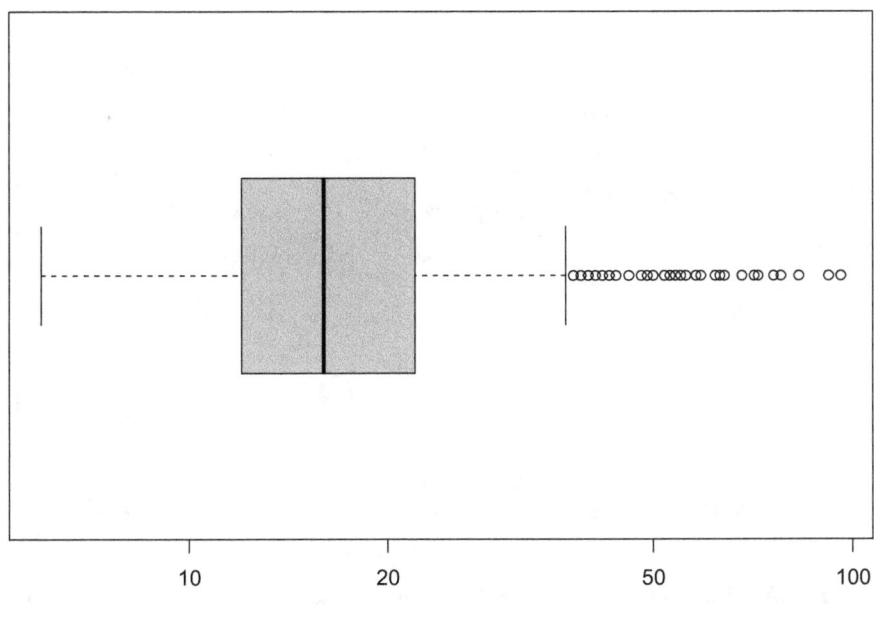

log Alanine transaminase (ALT) U/L (units per litre)

**Fig. 4.8.** Box plot of Alanine Transaminase (ALT) results from the SCAN dataset.

do this directly, but we need to select `log = "x"` if `horizontal = T` is used and `log = "y"` if `horizontal = F` (the default) (Figure 4.8).

```
boxplot(SCAN$alaninetrans,
log = "x",
horizontal = T,
xlab = "log Alanine transaminase (ALT) U/L
        (units per litre)")
```

### 4.3.4.2  *Example 2: A grouped box plot*

Box plots are particularly effective for showing variation between and within groups. This example shows haemoglobin test results from the SCAN dataset by age group (Figure 4.9). It is clear that haemoglobin declines with age but becomes more variable.

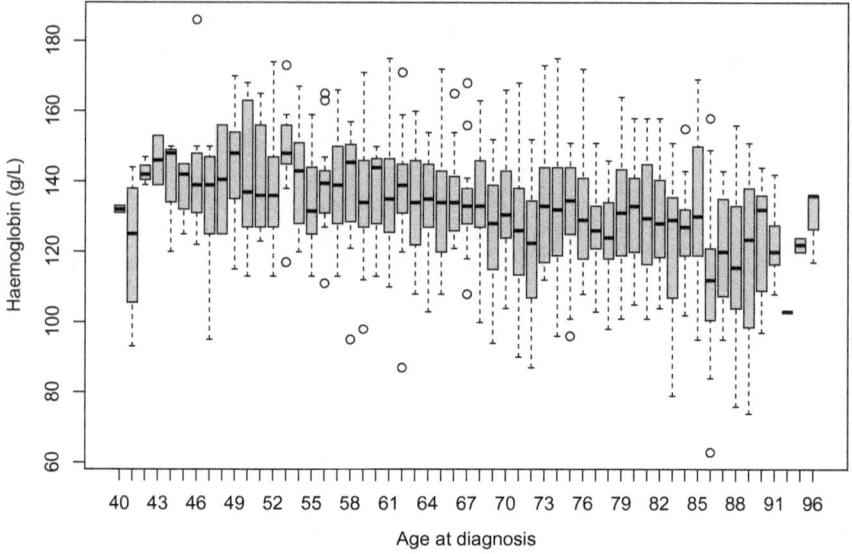

**Fig. 4.9.** Example of a grouped box plot: haemoglobin (g/L) by age group.

```
boxplot(HAEMRES ~ age,
data = SCAN,
ylab = "Haemoglobin (g/L)",
xlab = "Age at diagnosis")
```

### 4.3.5 *Comments*

The box plot is a relatively recent invention developed by John W. Tukey in the 1970s. Some variants have been proposed to add information on the display, including variable-width boxes, notched boxes, and a combination of the two (McGill *et al.*, 1978). The following code replicates the examples from the aforementioned paper. One is to add notches surrounding the medians and provide a measure of the significance of differences between the values, so that if the notches about two medians do not overlap, the medians are approximately significantly different at the 5% level. The variable-width box plot can add further information on the sample size in each box, with the width of each box being made proportional to the number of data points in the corresponding group.

```
# notches
boxplot(breaks ~ wool + tension,
data  = warpbreaks,
notch=T)

# variable width
frq <- xtabs(breaks ~ wool + tension,
data = warpbreaks)

# proportional to square root n
boxplot(breaks ~ wool + tension,
data  = warpbreaks,
boxwex = 0.05*sqrt(frq))
```

## 4.4   1-D scatter plot

### 4.4.1   *Overview*

One dimensional (1-D) scatter plots are a valuable alternative to box plots, particularly for diagnostic accuracy data. The `stripchart()` function can perform 1-D scatter plots for a single variable or by groups. With a bit of modification, the 1-D scatter plot can be an effective means of presentation.

### 4.4.2   *Data requirements*

The data supplied to the x argument should be ordinal or interval scale data. Grouped data can be accommodated using the formula syntax

```
stripchart(x ~ g)
```

where g is a vector identifying the different groups. Positioning of the groups can be controlled using the at argument (e.g., `stripchart(...,at = c(1.25,1.75))`, where the length of the vector is equal to the number of groups).

### 4.4.3  *Modifications*

#### 4.4.3.1  *Orientation*

For the stripchart, plots can be vertical or horizontal and selected using the `vertical` argument.

#### 4.4.3.2  *Point character adjustment*

Point characters or *plotting symbols* are selected using the `pch` option (Figure 4.10) or any single text character, e.g., `pch = "x"` or `pch = "+"`. Symbols corresponding to 21–25 allow the fill and background colours to be different using `col` and `bg` arguments respectively.

Point expansion is handled using the `cex` argument. Point expansion (`cex`) is the amount by which plotting text and symbols should be scaled relative to the default, where 1 is default, 1.5 is 50% larger, 0.5 is 50% smaller, etc. Data with same values will by default, be plotted on top of each other (`method = "overplot"`), but separating or *jittering* the points often creates more visual impact. The `method = "jitter"` argument moves the points by a random amount, separating points that would otherwise lie on top of one another. As jittering works by adding random noise (to the $x$ coordinate), it will change each time you do the plot; use `set.seed()` to retain precisely the same plot. The amount of jitter can be controlled using the `jitter` argument (e.g., `stripchart(..., jitter = 0.1, ...)`).

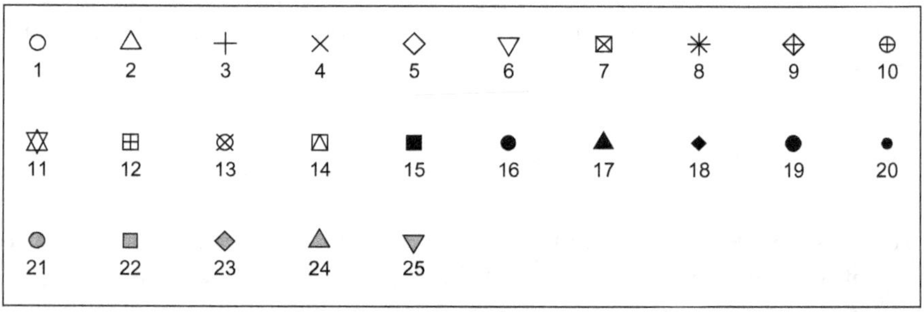

**Fig. 4.10.**  Point characters (plotting symbols) specified by the `pch` argument.

### 4.4.3.3 *Labelling*

Title and subtitles can be added to plots using the `main` and `sub` arguments. Axis labels, as per the other base R functions, are controlled using `xlab` and `ylab` arguments.

### 4.4.4 **Examples**

#### 4.4.4.1 *Example 1: Stripcharts – 1-D scatter*

The OXFIT dataset contains blood test results from patients referred for rapid investigation for colorectal cancer. Figure 4.11 shows scatter of results in the patients later found not to have cancer.

```
data(OXFIT, package = "R4HCR")
stripchart(fit_val ~ cancer,
data = OXFIT,
pch = 19,
cex=0.5,
method="jitter",
col = "gray40",
xlab = expression(paste("FIT (",mu,"g/Hb faeces)")),
ylab = c("Not CRC","CRC")
)
```

Jittering the points allows us to see the slightly unusual clustering of results at around 450 ($\mu$g/Hb faeces), resulting from the lab truncating some of the values higher than 450.

## 4.5   2-D scatter plot

### 4.5.1 *Overview*

Usually, a 'scatter plot' refers to a plot of two variables – a two-dimensional (2-D) scatter plot. A scatter plot is a good way to show how two quantities vary together and is used widely in statistics. The choice of which variable to put on which axis is not always obvious, but if one of the variables can be thought of as the outcome or response variable, we would usually put this on the (vertical) $y$-axis and the explanatory variable on the (horizontal) $x$-axis.

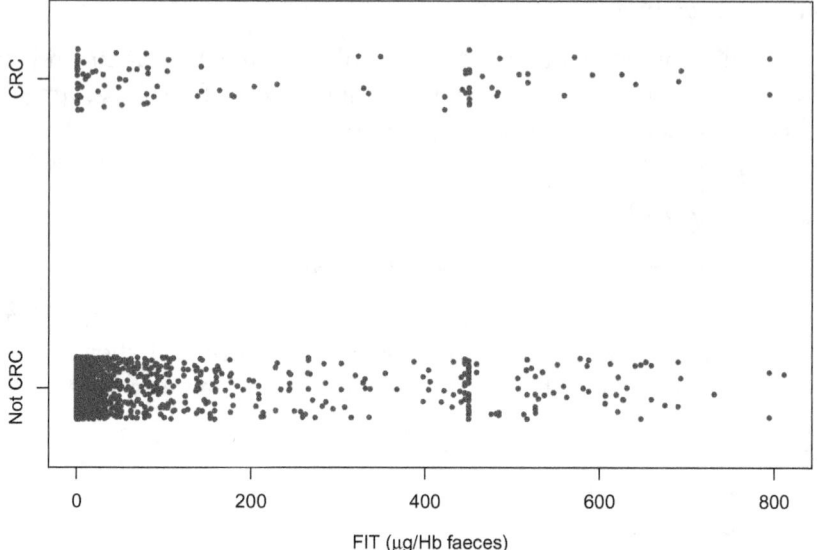

**Fig. 4.11.** Strip chart (with jittering) of FIT levels in patients with and without colorectal cancer (CRC).

### 4.5.2 *Data requirements*

The preferred base R function for drawing a 2-D scatter plot for two continuous variables is simply `plot()`. There are many plot methods for different R objects and functions, so when you call `plot()`, the result depends on what type of object is supplied. If `x` and `y` are vectors of equal length, then `plot(x,y)` will return a two-dimensional scatter plot (actually called `plot.default`). If the `x` coordinate is not given, the function will revert to plotting `y` against an index from 1 to length `y`. If `x` is the result of a linear model (`x <- lm()`), then the `plot(x)` will produce a series of diagnostic plots relating to the linear model fit. If `x` is a table with two or more dimensions, then `plot(x)` will produce a mosaic plot. There are over 50 plot functions to date (use `methods(plot)` to see them all).

### 4.5.3 *Plot types*

There are nine different plot types to choose from (see Figure 4.12).

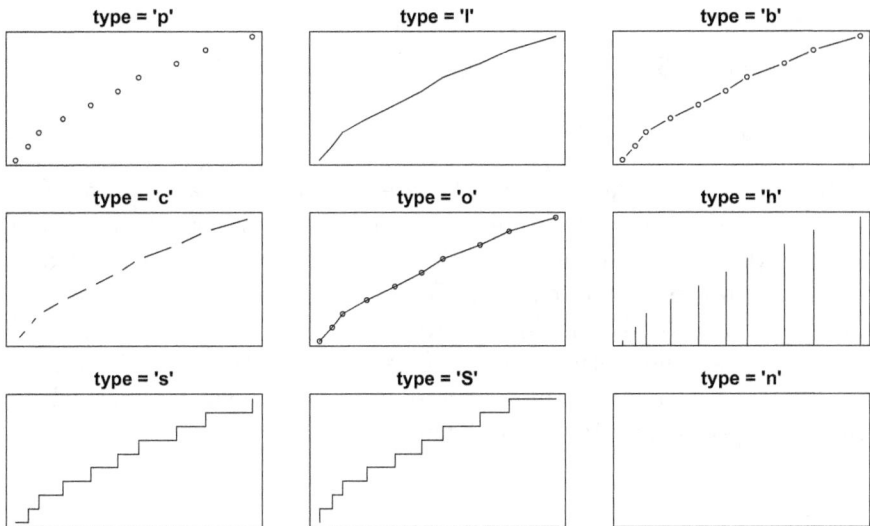

**Fig. 4.12.** Plot type options in `plot()`, 'p' for points, 'l' for lines, 'b' for both, 'c' for the lines part alone of 'b', 'o' for both 'overplotted', 'h' for 'histogram'-like vertical lines, 's' for stair steps, 'S' for other steps, and 'n' for no plotting.

### 4.5.3.1 *Axes*

Axes can be removed altogether using the `axes = F` option, and the *x*-axis and *y*-axis tick marks suppressed using the `xaxt = "n"` and `yaxt = "n"` options, respectively. Logarithmic scale axes, which can be very helpful in showing multiplicative relationships, can be selected using the `log = "y"` or `log = "x"` options.

```
# y transformed using natural log.
plot(x,y, log = "y")

# x and y transformed using natural log.
plot(x,y, log = "xy")
```

These will be natural logarithms, and the tick mark labels will be in the original units. Logarithms to other bases will need to be coded manually.

### 4.5.3.2   *Legends*

See Section 4.2.3.4.

### 4.5.3.3   *Annotating the plot*

Annotating the basic scatter plot is easy once you know how. One common task involves adding additional lines, either as fitted lines to the existing data or as extra data. To add another batch of data to an existing plot, you can use the `lines()` command to add lines and `points()` to add the data as point characters. Adding a linear-fit line is quite straightforward using the `abline()` command. Generally, for two continuous variables, $x$ and $y$, and a linear model with an intercept, you would do the following:

```
plot(x,y)
abline(reg = lm(y ~ x))
```

Vertical or horizontal lines can also be added using `abline()`.

```
abline(h = 0, lty = 2) # dashed horizontal line at y = 0
abline(v = 5, lty = 2) # dashed vertical lines at x = 5
abline(a, b, ...) # generic line for a + bx
```

The functions `lines()` and `segments()` can also be used to add lines to plots (see Section 4.7.4.2) – the segments function gives more flexibility. Text can be added using the `text()` command, e.g., `text (x = 1, y= 1, labels = "some text")` after the initial plot call. The function `polygon()` draws the polygons corresponding to vertices given in $x$ and $y$. This function adds confidence regions (see Example 4.7.4.3) and shaded areas on plots. It can be tricky to get this correct (particularly for curves), and it pays to know how to generate sequences and which built-in functions can help with the $x$–$y$ coordinates.

### 4.5.4   *Examples*

#### 4.5.4.1   *Example 1: Two continuous variables*

We illustrate a 2-D scatter plot using mean cell haemoglobin and mean cell volume from the OXFIT dataset (Figure 4.13). We add

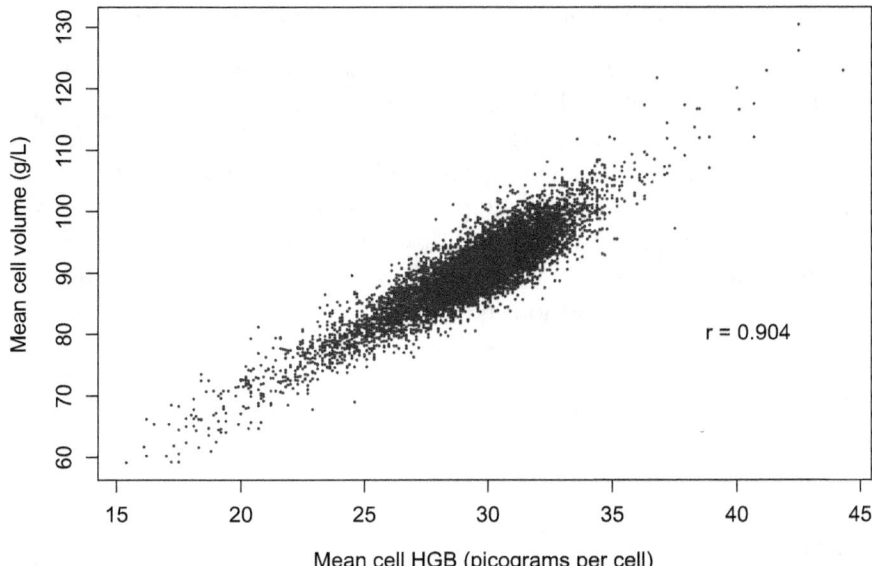

**Fig. 4.13.** Scatter plot of mean cell haemoglobin and mean cell volume.

to the plot the estimated (Pearson) correlation coefficient using the
`text()` command after first estimating the correlation using the
`cor()` function. The plot clearly shows that they are strongly positively correlated.

```
plot(mean_cell_vol ~ mean_cell_hgb,
data = OXFIT,
subset = cancer ==0,
cex = 0.3,
pch = 16,
col = "gray30",
xlab = "Mean cell HGB (picograms per cell)",
ylab = "Mean cell volume (g/L)")
fit.cor <- cor(FITnormal$mean_cell_hgb,
FITnormal$mean_cell_vol)
text(x = 40,y = 80,
labels = paste0("r = ",
format(fit.cor,nsmall=2,digits=3)),
cex = 0.8)
```

4.5.4.2   *Example 2: Two continuous variables with smoother*

We will sometimes want to add a non-parametric smoothing trend
line to a scatter plot. This is the kind of task that is made very simple
through packages such as **ggplot2**, but it is not difficult using base
R once you know how. Doing more of the work yourself gives you
more control and may also help you understand how it is derived.
We use a subset of the OXFIT dataset to demonstrate this. To add a
non-parametric smoother to a standard scatter plot, we can use the
**scatter.smooth()** function, e.g.,

```
# create subset of OXFIT data
OXFIT_small <- OXFIT[1:999,]

# a scatter plot with smoothing spline overlaid
scatter.smooth(x,y)
```

However, adding confidence bands to the plot takes more work.
The key is to use the **predict()** function in combination with
the **loess()** function and to specify **se = T** to get the estimated
standard errors. We can then use these to draw bands around
the smoothing lines corresponding to the 95% confidence limits
(see Figure 4.14). Alternatively, we could add a band of trans-
parent colour around the smoothing line using the **polygon()**
function.

```
# take a subset of rows.
pdata <- OXFIT[1:999,]

# sort the data by the 'x' variable
pdata <- pdata[order(pdata$haemoglobin),]

y <- pdata$mean_cell_hgb
x <- pdata$haemoglobin
```

```
plot(y ~ x,
     data = pdata,
     cex = 0.4,
     col = "gray50",
     xlab = "Haemoglobin (g/L)",
     ylab = "Mean cell Hgb (picograms per cell)")

# loess fit smoother with standard error
smth <- predict(loess(y ~ x), se=T)

# smooth fit (middle line)
smfit <- smth$fit

# lower and upper band
lb <- smfit - qt(0.975,smth$df)*smth$se
ub <- smfit + qt(0.975,smth$df)*smth$se
```

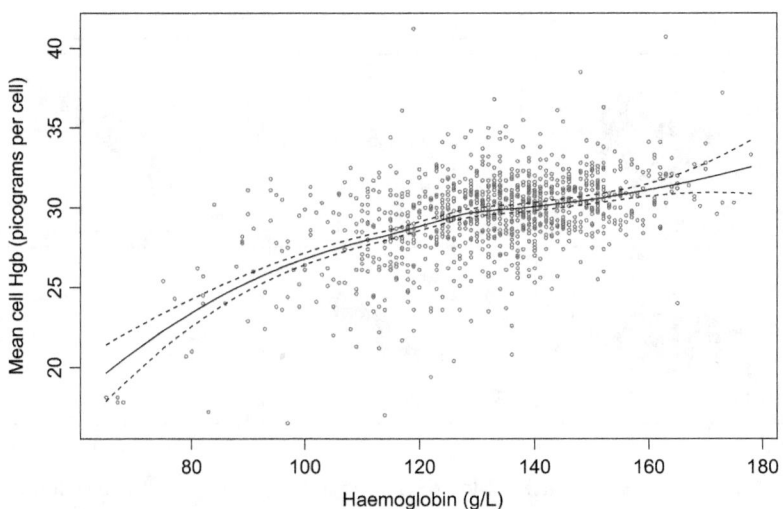

**Fig. 4.14.**  Scatter plot of mean cell haemoglobin (Hgb) and haemoglobin, with smoother (solid line) and lower and upper confidence bands (dashed lines).

```
# add lines to the plot
lines(x,smfit)
lines(x, lb, lty=2)
lines(x, ub, lty=2)
```

To draw a polygon in R, you need to supply the x and y coordinates corresponding to each of the corners of the shape you want to plot. The coordinates can be ordered clockwise or counter-clockwise and start from any corner of the shape. To add colour with transparency you will need to supply the colour in 'RGB' format.

### 4.5.4.3 Example 3: A matrix of scatter plots

To produce a matrix of scatter plots, use the function `pairs(x, ...)`, where x is a matrix or data frame (see Figure 4.15).

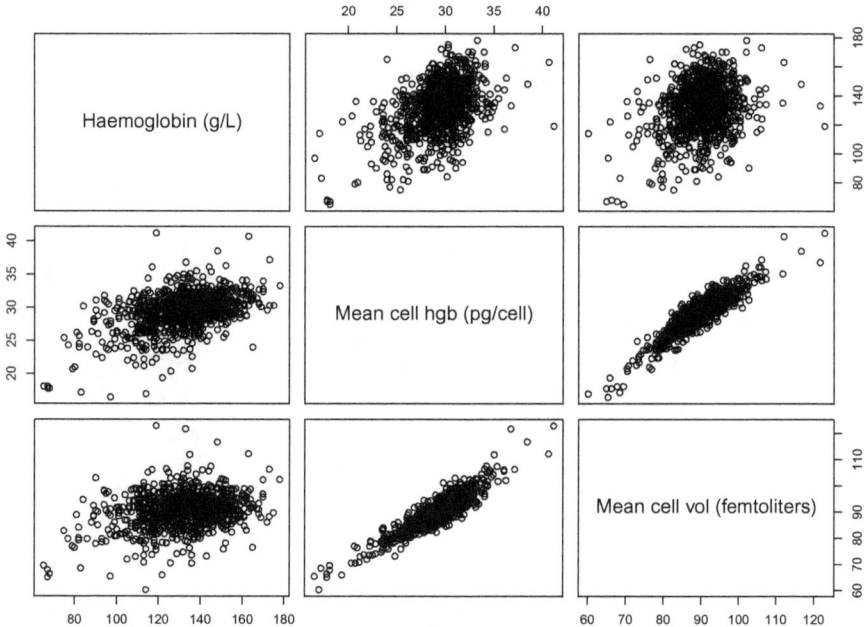

**Fig. 4.15.** A matrix scatter plot of haemoglobin, mean cell haemoglobin, and mean cell volume.

```
X <- subset(pdata,
select = c("haemoglobin","mean_cell_hgb",
"mean_cell_vol"))
pairs(X)
```

## 4.6 Probability or Q–Q plot

### 4.6.1 *Overview*

Probability of quantile-quantile (Q–Q) plots are used to help identity outliers, and also as a visual check of the goodness of fit to a reference probability distribution. The plot compares the quantiles of the observed data against a reference line drawn from theoretical quantiles from a known probability distribution. The observed data can be said to be consistent with the reference probability distribution if the majority of the data falls on, or close to the reference line, and inconsistent if the data deviates significantly from the line. Points far from the line usually correspond to outliers or unusual values. A general method for comparing a sample $x$ with theoretical quantiles from any distribution consists of the following steps:

(1) Calculate probability points for data $x$ using `ppoints(x)`.
(2) Calculate the theoretical quantiles for these probabilities for the distribution you want to compare to (e.g., for the normal, do `qnorm(ppoints(x))`).
(3) Plot these against the (sorted) data.
(4) (Optional) Assess straightness by plotting a straight line through two probability points (normally the upper and lower quartiles). Use the `qqline()` function for this.

For normal Q–Q plots we can just use the `qqplot()` and `qqline()` functions.

### 4.6.2 *Data requirements*

This method can be used with continuous, discrete, and rank data.

### 4.6.3   *Modifications*

By default, `qqline()` and `qqnorm()` put the sample data on the *y*-axis and the theoretical quantiles on the *x*-axis. This can be switched by changing the default `datax = F` to `datax = T`.

### 4.6.4   *Examples*

#### 4.6.4.1   *Example 1: A normal probability plot*

We simulate data from a non-normal distribution (with heavy positive skew) and then see if the `qqnorm()` plot can detect the mismatch of distributions (Figure 4.16).

```
# simulated data from an exponential distribution
x <- rexp(100,1)
qqnorm(x, datax = T, main = NULL)
qqline(x, datax = T)
```

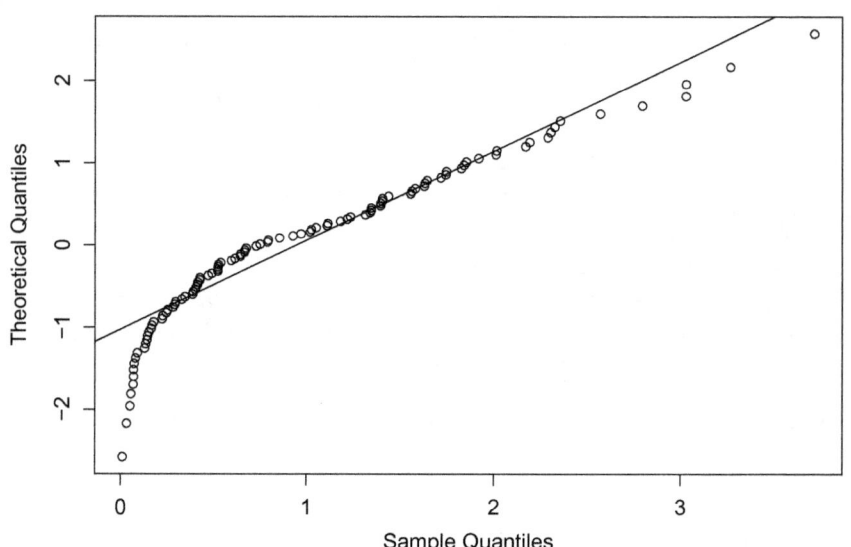

**Fig. 4.16.**   An example of a normal quantile–quantile (Q–Q) plot fitted to positively skewed data.

### 4.6.4.2 *Example 2: Log-normal probability plot*

We now assess the normality assumption for the platelet data in the OXFIT dataset. We start with a normal probability plot and then assess whether the data are more consistent with a log-normal distribution. If $w$ is distributed normally then $x = \exp(w)$ has a log-normal distribution. Hence, we can log-transform the platelet data using the normal probability plot as before.

```
x <- OXFIT$platelets
qqnorm(x, main = "Normal")
qqline(x)
w <- log(OXFIT$platelets)
qqnorm(w, main = "Log-normal")
axis(4)
qqline(w)
```

The systematic deviation from the line at the northeast corner of the normal probability plot would suggest a long tail and evidence that the assumption of normality would not be justified. The log-normal plot has the opposite problem (Figure 4.17).

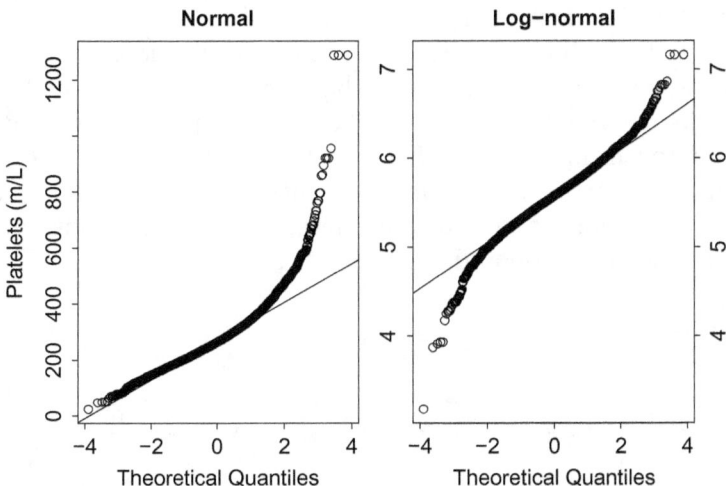

**Fig. 4.17.** Normal Q–Q plot (left panel) and log-normal Q–Q plot (right panel) of the platelet data from the OXFIT study.

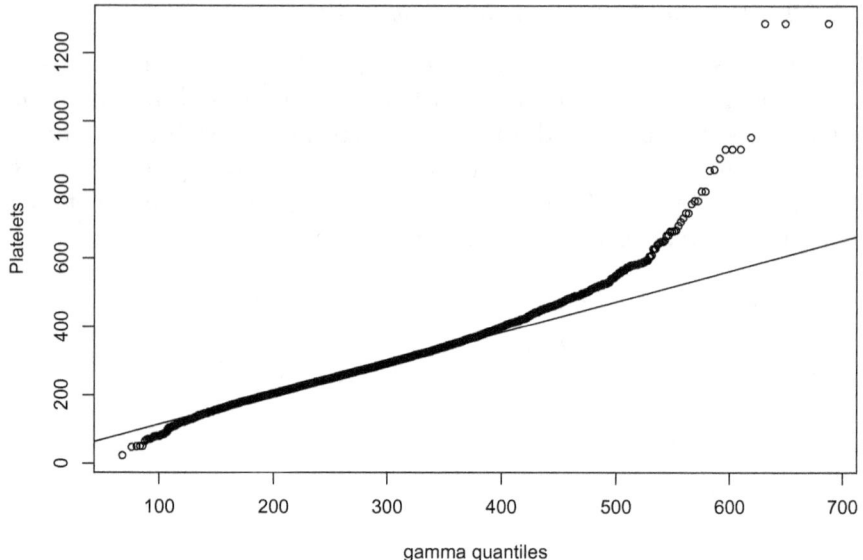

**Fig. 4.18.**  A Q–Q plot of the platelet data against a gamma distribution.

### 4.6.4.3  *Example 3: A probability plot for any distribution*

The steps in Section 4.6.4.1 can be generalised to any distribution. One extra step will be required. For other distributions, we may need to provide parameters. Some, like the t and chi-square distributions, require degrees of freedom, while others require parameters that must be estimated from the data. For example, if we wanted to compare the platelet data to a gamma distribution we would first have to estimate the shape and rate parameters for a gamma distribution (see the following code and Figure 4.18).

```
x <- sort(OXFIT$platelets)

# Estimate the parameters of the gamma distribution
(parms <- MASS::fitdistr(x, "gamma"))

# calculate the quantiles
qs <- qgamma(ppoints(x),
shape = parms$estimate[1],
```

```
rate = parms$estimate[2])

# plot the sorted data against the quantiles
plot(qs,x,
cex = 0.8,
xlab = "gamma quantiles",
ylab = "Platelets (m/L)")

# Add a reference line
qqline(x,
distribution = function(p)
qgamma(p,shape = parms$estimate[1],
rate = parms$estimate[2]))
```

```
##        shape            rate
##    1.229376e+01    4.482821e-02
##    (1.708831e-01) (6.358341e-04)
```

The platelet data does not conform to either a normal, log-normal or gamma distribution. In our experience, it is not uncommon to encounter data that does not conform to any regular probability distributions. But the Q–Q plot has helped to quickly reach this conclusion.

## 4.7   Building a plot from scratch

In the previous sections, we showed the code required to draw several *high-level* basic plot types. We now look at low-level plotting functions that allow finer control over each element of the graph or figure. The functions are, again, all part of the basic R installation, keeping with our general philosophy of R programming. There are external packages that offer some incredible functions for drawing graphs (notably, the **ggplot2** package), and we encourage the reader to seek these out. However, it may be surprising to find what can be done with just base R. The trade-off for this level of control is that we will need to do more coding than is strictly necessary, but this often pays off if we need to make precise adjustments to the figure later. The modular approach to building graphs using low-level functions involves the following steps;

(1) Set global options, e.g., the plotting region and margins.
(2) Start a new plot frame or window.
(3) Set the coordinate system for a graphics window, e.g., the axes limits.
(4) Add axes, tick marks, frames, and the foreground colour.
(5) Add data points, lines, and symbols.
(6) Add annotations, e.g., arrows, shading, and contextual information.
(7) Add legends and titles.

### 4.7.1   *Setting global options*

Global options apply across the current R session, unless specified. Setting global graphical parameters can make the process of modifying plots simpler and quicker. For example, if we wanted to reduce the point character size across a series of plots, we need only change the global point size parameter once, rather than modifying multiple lines of code.

#### 4.7.1.1   *Graphical parameters*

The list of parameters and their current values can be accessed by typing **par()** – there are 72 in total! It can make sense to save the current values so that you can undo any changes you make without starting a new R session. We do this by creating an object called **defaultPar**.

```
defaultPar <- par() # default values saved
defaultPar$cex

# change globally all point cex to 0.8
par(cex = 0.8)
par()['cex']

# change back
par <- defaultPar
par['cex'] <- defaultPar$cex
par['cex']
```

### 4.7.1.2 *Plot layout*

The default layout in R is for a single plot. We tend to use the
`mfrow()` option to put more than one plot into a device window. This
option takes an argument of the form `c(no.rows, no.columns)`,
with subsequent figures drawn row-wise. To set a panel plot with
one row and two columns, we would do

```
par(mfrow = c(1,2))

# 1st plot is placed in row 1, column 1

# 2nd plot is placed in row 1, column 2.
```

When we have multiple plotting regions on one page, we might
want to adjust the size of the margins; we can do this with either the
`mar` option for the number of lines of margin to be specified on the
four sides of the plot or `mai`, which gives the margin size specified in
inches. The order of the margins is shown in Figure 4.19.

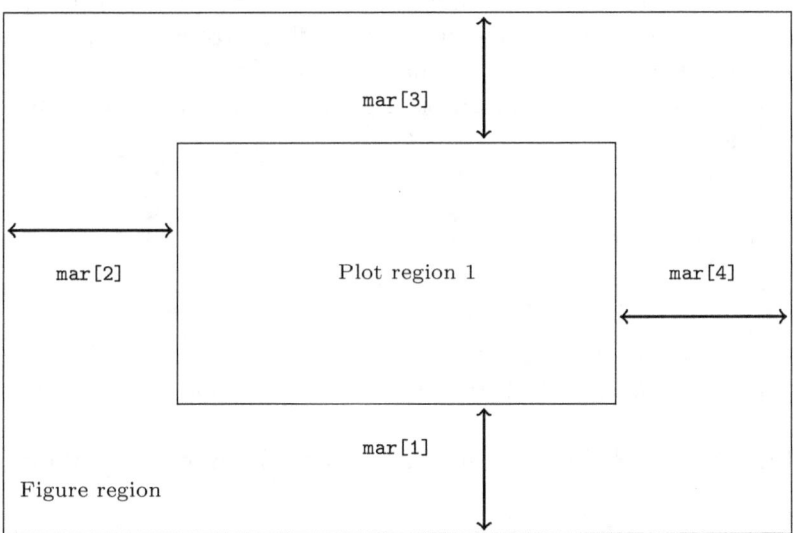

**Fig. 4.19.** The figure and plot region with the order of margins.

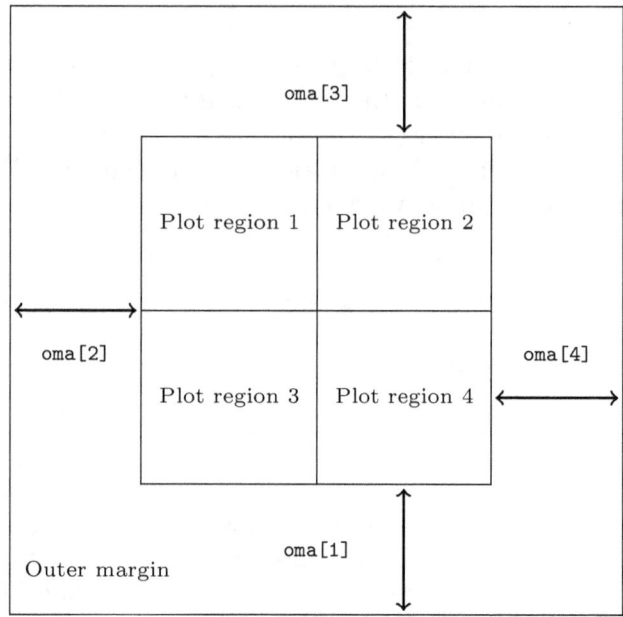

**Fig. 4.20.** The R plot regions and outer margins. *Plot order depends on* mfrow(2,2).

The default margins in lines (mar) is c(5,4,4,2) + 0.1. The order of starting at the bottom and moving around the plot clockwise is the same for the outer margins (see Figure 4.20). For example, to reduce the top margin to 2.1 lines rather than 4.1 lines, we would do

```
# default is
par('mar')
```

```
## [1] 5.1 4.1 4.1 2.1
```

```
# this sets new margins
par(mar = c(5.1,4.1,2.1,2.1))
```

Similarly, to reduce an outer margin to the plot, we could do.

```
# outer margins in lines of text.
par(oma = c(0.1,0.1,0.1,0.1))
```

```
# outer margins in inches.
par(omi = c(0.05,0.05,0.05,0.05))

#  outer margins as a fraction (in [0, 1][0,1])
# of the device region.
par(omd)
```

### 4.7.2   *Setting the coordinates*

Next, set the coordinates of the graphics window using the
plot.window() function. The limits of the $x$ and $y$ axis are specified using the xlim and ylim options.

```
plot.window(xlim = c(0,1), ylim = c(0,1))
```

Axes can be added using the **axis()** commands. Use the
side = 1 for below, side = 2 for left, side = 3 for above, and
side = 4 for right positioning. The at argument gives the points
at which tick-marks are to be drawn, the labels are the text placed
at the tick points.

```
# Add axes to right hand side
axis(4, at = c(1,2,3), labels = c("fee","fi","fo"))
```

You can set the background colour by doing, for example, **par**
(bg = "gray60"). A frame can be added using

```
box(col = "grey60")
```

and foreground colour can be added with **rect()**

```
rect(xleft = par("usr")[1],
ybottom = par("usr")[3],
xright = par("usr")[2],
ytop = par("usr")[4],
col = "gray96")
```

The **rect()** function draws a rectangle at given coordinates. In this example we set coordinates that correspond to the extremes of the plotting region by using the **par()** function. To add a grid, we could do

```
grid(col = "white")
```

The **grid()** function works well when the axes tick marks follow the default, but we have found that this function does not always align with the tick marks, especially when we set custom tick marks. When this is the case, it is better to use the **abline()** or **segments()** function, as this offers finer control of the horizontal and vertical positions. Assuming that the tick marks for both the $x$ and $y$ axes are stored in vectors called **xsq** and **ysq**, respectively, the following code will produce the grid at the correct position:

```
# Use axTicks() function to position grid lines

xsq <- axTicks(side = 1)
ysq <- axTicks(side = 2)

# create grid using abline()
abline(h = ysq, v = xsq,
col = "lightgray", lty = "dotted")
```

### 4.7.3   Adding data

Data in the form of points, lines, smoothers, etc., can be added once the window has been defined. To add points, use the **points()** function.

```
points(x, s1, pch = 21, bg = "gray80")
```

and for lines use **lines()**.

```
lines(x,y,lty = 2, col = "gray60")
```

These can be combined or added to in virtually any form, which makes this a very flexible way to build graphics. A spline or curve can be drawn using the **xspline()** function.

```
# An example from Murrell,P. R Graphics
plot.new()
plot.window(xlim =c(-1,1), ylim = c(-1,1))
box()
t <- seq(60,360,30)
x <- cos(t/180*pi)*t/360
y <- sin(t/180*pi)*t/360
xspline(x,y,shape= 1)
points(x,y,pch = 16)
```

### 4.7.4 Annotating the plot

There are many functions in base R to annotate plots.

#### 4.7.4.1 Arrows

To add an arrow to a base R plot, use the **arrows()** function. The position of one end of the arrow is controlled using the x0 and y0 arguments, and the other end with x1 and y1. The arrowhead size is controlled using the **length** argument, while its angle is modified using **angle**. Use the **code** option to select one of three arrow types: if **code = 1**, an arrowhead is drawn at x0,y0, whereas if **code = 2**, an arrowhead is drawn at x1,y1, and for arrowheads drawn at both ends, select **code = 3**.

```
arrows(x0 = 0.05,
y0 = 0.9,
x1 = 0.45,
y1 = 0.9,
length = 0.05,
angle = 45,
code = 3)
```

The **arrows()** function can also be used to draw confidence intervals (lines and staples) by setting the angle to zero.

#### 4.7.4.2 Segments

The **segments()** function allows finer control over the drawing of lines than **lines()** or **abline()**. The position of the lines is controlled similarly to the **arrows()** function with x0,y0,x1,y1 coordinates, but these can be single numbers or vectors, which can facilitate drawing many lines in one go.

```
# drawing a series of lines
segments(x0 = rep(0.5,5),
y0 = seq(0.5,0.6,0.02),
x1 = rep(0.6,5),
y1 = seq(0.5,0.6,0.02),
col= 'gray40')
```

### 4.7.4.3  Generic shapes

Practically any shape can be drawn using the **polygon()** function, but there are other functions to add shapes to plots, including the **rect()** and **symbols()** functions.

```
# A rectangle
rect(xleft = 0.05,
ybottom = 0.45,
xright = 0.4,
ytop = 0.2,
density = 10,
angle = 45)

# A triangle
polygon(x = c(0.65,0.85,0.75),
y = c(0.2,0.2,0.4))

# A circle
symbols(x = 2, y = 12, circles = 0.3,add=T)

# thermometers?
symbols(x = 0.5,
y = 0.5,
thermometers = cbind(.5, 1, 0.1),
inches = .5, fg = 2)
```

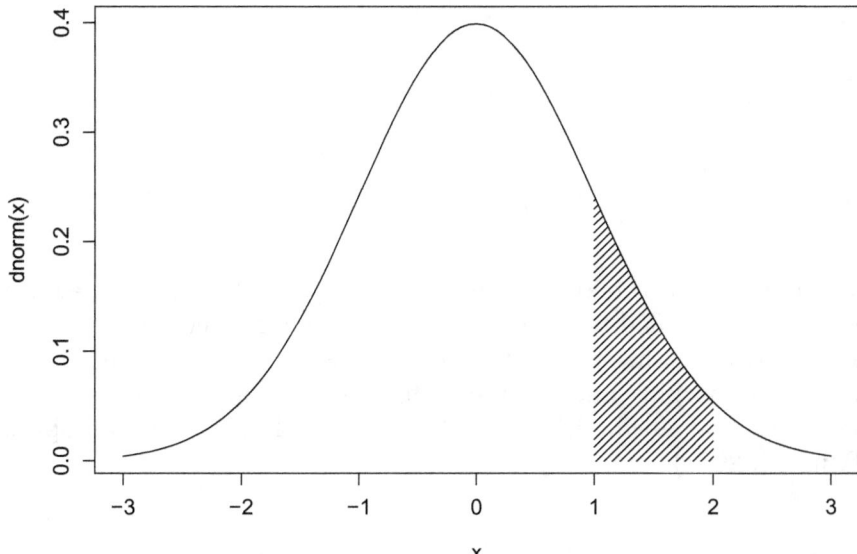

**Fig. 4.21.** Normal density plot with area between $x = 1$ and $x = 2$, shaded using the `polygon()` function.

The `polygon` function is particularly helpful for shading tail areas on density plots (see Figure 4.21).

```
curve(dnorm,from = -3, to = 3)
xs <- c(1,seq(1,2,0.01),2)
ys <- c(0,dnorm(seq(1,2,0.01)),0)
polygon(x = xs,y = ys,border = F, density = 20)
```

#### 4.7.4.4 *Adding text*

The size and appearance of text in a plot can be controlled in several ways. Absolute text size can be set using **par(ps = 12))** and a multiplier **cex = 1**, either globally or within a text command.

```
text("Some text",x = 0.5, y= 0.5, cex = 0.9)
```

Font type and family can be set using the **font** and **family()** arguments.

```
text("Bold",...,font = 2)
text("Italic",...,font = 3)
text("Bold Italic",...,font = 4)
text("mono", ..., family = "mono")
text("serif", ..., family = "serif")
text("sans", ..., family = "sans")
```

Justification of text is set using the `adj` option, with `adj=0` producing left-justified text, `adj = 1` producing right-justified text, and `adj = 0.5` centring the text. Rotating text can be set using `srt`. In the outer margins and high-level figures, text may only be drawn at angles that are multiples of 90°, controlled using the `las` option (Murrell, 2011).

```
# left justified text, at 20 degree
text("Some text",...,adj = 0, srt = 20)
```

Adding math expressions to plots can be done using **expression** alone or in combination with **paste()**. Use **bquote()** for partial substitution in expressions and for combining mathematical annotation and R objects. The following code chunk provides some examples of the use of both functions:

```
# Units
expression("("~degree*C*")") # degrees celcius

expression(paste("(",mu,"g/L)")) # microgram/L

# math notation
expression(x %+-% y)     # plus minus
expression(y^2)          # superscript.
expression(sqrt(x))      # square root
expression(sqrt(x, y))   # yth root of x
expression(hat(x))       # circumflex
```

```
expression(bar(x))        # x bar
expression(x %*% y)       # times symbol
expression(x[i])          # subscript
expression(infinity)      # infinity symbol
expression(frac(x, y))    # fraction

# Combinations
expression(bar(x)==sum(frac(x[i], n),i==1,n))

# Greek letters
expression(paste(hat(beta)/2))
expression(mu == 0)

# combining plot math and saved objects
# m is scalar
bquote(bar(x) == .(m))
```

#### 4.7.4.5 *Titles and axes labels*

The **titles**() command allows you to add $x$-axis and $y$-axis labels as well as main titles and subtitles to a plot, e.g.,

```
title(main = "This is a title")
title(sub = "This is a subtitle")
title(xlab = "X axis label at line 2 spacing",line = 2)
title(ylab = "Y axis label at line 0 spacing", line = 0)
```

If you want to add axis labels to the right-hand side or the top of the graph, you can do this using

```
mtext(text = "Right hand side axes label",
side=4, line = 0.5)
```

For legends, see Section 4.2.3.4.

### 4.7.5   *A template*

Putting this altogether, we have

```r
par(mfrow = c(1,1),  # plot(s) playout
mar = c(5.1,4.1,4.1,2.1), # b,l,t,r margin (in lines)
oma = c(4,4,2,2),   # outer margins (in lines)
cex.axis = 0.9, # magnification for axis annotation
cex = 0.8, # magnification for symbols
...
)

# plot region
plot.new()
plot.window(xlim=c(),ylim=c())
rect(par("usr"),
par("usr")[3],
par("usr")[2],
par("usr")[4],
col = "white") # filled box
box(col = "grey60") # outline

# data
points(x,y)    # add points and/or lines
lines(x,y)    # draw single lines

# annotation
axis(side = 1)    # 1=bottom, 2=left, 3=top, 4=right
arrows(x0, y0,x1,y1)
text(x,y,labels)
rect(xleft, ybottom,xright,ytop)
segments(x0, y0, x1, y1)  # useful for multiple lines
polygon(x ,y)
abline(a,b,h,v)  # draw vertical/horizontal/sloped lines

# legend
legend(x = ,
```

```
y = 0.5,
legend = c("series 1", "series 2",...),
col = "black",
lty = c(1,1,...),
pch = c(1,2,...),
ncol = 1,
inset = 0.05,
bty = "y",
cex=0.85,
title="A title",
text.font = 3,
bg='gray95')

# titles
main(title, xlab, ylab)
mtext(x = ,y = ) # margin text
```

## 4.8 Exporting graphs

Graphs can be exported directly from an IDE, such as RStudio, but it is easy to save images and files using syntax. This makes the process quicker if you need to make changes to the plot and allows control of the resolution and size of the graphic. BMP, JPEG, PNG, and TIFF format bitmap files, as well as PDFs, are supported. The key to using these commands is to sandwich the plot code between a graphics device function, e.g., **png()** and **dev.off()**.

```
png(file = "myplot.png")
plot(1:10)
...
dev.off()

# landscape pdf plot
pdf("mydir.pdf",paper = "USr")
plot(...)
dev.off()
```

```
# 300 dpi, wider
png("MyFigure.png", res = 300,
width = 2200*1.3, height = 2200)
```

## 4.9   Problems and exercises

(1) Use the `biopsy` data from the `MASS` package to draw a side-by-side bar plot of clump thickness by tumour class (benign or maligant). Try using the `xtabs()` function to prepare the data.

(2) Use the `lung` data from the `survival` package.

   (a) Produce a *true* histogram of survival time. Set the breaks to be the square root of survival times. Describe the distribution. Are there any outliers?

   (b) Add a kernal-density line to the plot.

   (c) Generate a box plot to show the distribution of calorie consumption at meals according to age group. Are there any outliers?

   (d) Add the raw data to the box plot using `stripchart()`, jittering the points to help clearly show the volume of data.

   (e) Make a bar plot of ECOG performance score by sex. Produce stacked and unstacked versions of the bar plot.

   (f) Add numbers to the bars to indicate frequency counts within each category.

   (g) Write down the syntax that will export the bar graph to a PDF.

   (h) Create a Cleveland's dot plot of the Karnofsky performance score as rated by patients by age group and sex. This plot can be done using the `dotchart()` function. Start by reading the help page and run the example given at the bottom of the help page. You can use the `tapply` function to obtain summary statistics for each subclass.

(3) The `Pima.tr` dataset from the `MASS` package includes data from women, who were at least 21 years old, of Pima Indian heritage, and living near Phoenix, Arizona. The women were tested for diabetes according to World Health Organization criteria. This

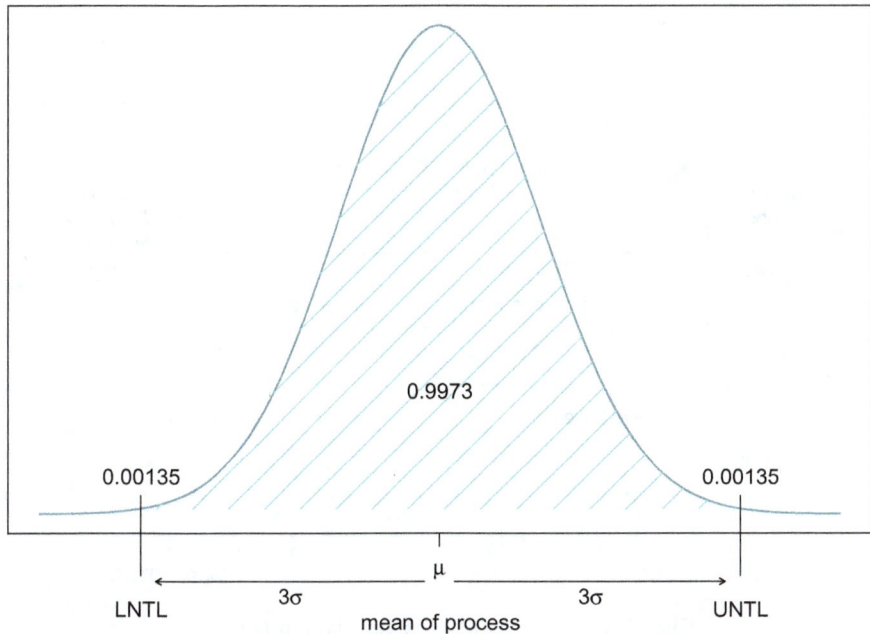

**Fig. 4.22.** Upper and lower natural tolerance (UNTL and LNTL) limits around the process mean.

version of the dataset contains a randomly selected set of 200 subjects (`Pima.te` contains the remaining 332 subjects). Generate a scatter plot of triceps skin fold thickness and body mass index with a smoothing line added. Check the plot and make any necessary adjustments.

(a) Adapt the previous plot so that the $y$-axis label includes the units for BMI, including a superscript of '2' for metres squared.

(4) Using a modular approach, recreate in whole or in part Figure 4.22, which illustrates the principle of upper and lower natural tolerance (UNTL and LNTL) limits around the process mean in measurement system analysis.

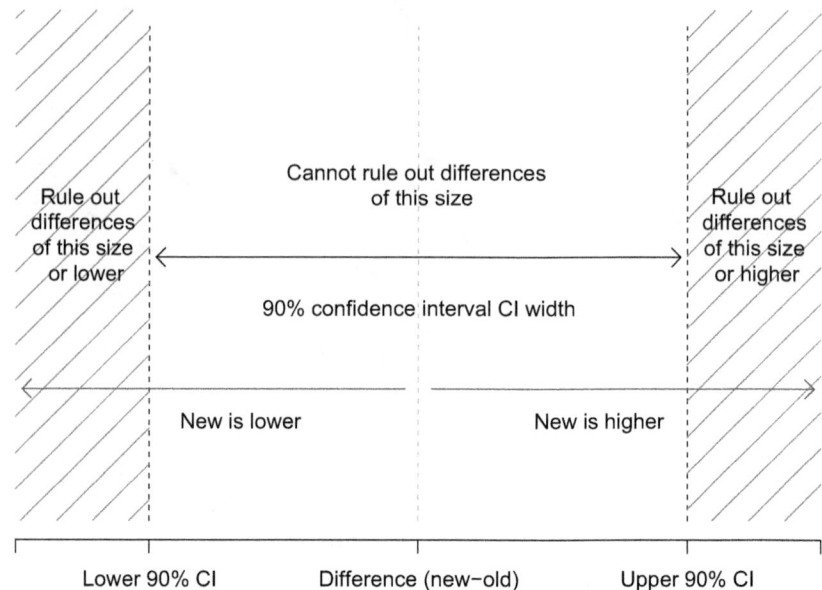

**Fig. 4.23.** The equivalence testing procedure.

(5) Using a modular approach, recreate Figure 4.23, which illustrates the equivalence testing procedure.

# Chapter 5

# Statistical tests for comparing two samples

Comparing outcomes between two *samples* of data is common in healthcare research. Typically, the samples are from two *independent* groups of patients or two samples from the same patients. Outcomes may be physiological parameters, scales, or clinical events. In this chapter, we show how to compare two samples of interval, binary, and categorical outcome data.

**Objectives and learning outcomes**

The objectives for this chapter are to:

- outline the fundamental consideration in choosing a method of analysis
- apply the principles of estimation and hypothesis testing to comparing groups of observations for different types of data
- introduce both parametric and non-parametric approaches to analysis

After reading this chapter, you should be able to:

- use R to carry out appropriate statistical tests for comparing two samples of continuous and categorical data
- interpret the results of statistical analyses, such as hypothesis tests, $p$-values, and confidence intervals
- understand the difference between statistical significance and clinical importance

## 5.1    Considerations

Choosing the correct statistical test can sometimes be challenging. Working through the following steps will help you determine which test is the most appropriate and which R function should be used.

### 5.1.1    *Data types*

The first consideration should be the type of data. For categorical data, only a limited set of tests are applicable, whereas for interval scale data, a wide range of options exists, one of which involves collapsing the data into categories. In the case of binary data, we should also ask: are we comparing rates or proportions? If the data are proportions, the next question is whether we should compare differences in proportions, relative risks, or odds ratios.

### 5.1.2    *Sample size*

The sample size being tested should factor into your decision-making when selecting a statistical test. For example, the $t$ test is suitable for small and large sample sizes, but the $z$ test should be reserved for large samples (as a rough guide here, assume large means $n > 100$ in each group). With categorical data, one should pay attention to the numbers within each cell of the table rather than the overall sample size. For example, the large sample chi-square test for binary data will display an error if one or more of the *expected* cell counts is $\leq 5$.

### 5.1.3    *Independent or related samples*

We need to understand how the data were collected and determine whether the two samples are from *independent* or *non-independent* groups. In what is occasionally termed the A/B design, patients are divided (often through randomisation) into two groups (A and B). As these groups in this study design consist of different individuals (one individual cannot be in both groups), the samples are considered independent. Conversely, if the same individuals are assessed on two occasions or if the two samples involve patients who have been paired in some manner, they are regarded as non-independent, or *paired*. Tests such as the *t* test can be used for both independent and non-independent settings, but you will have to select the appropriate version for your data.

### 5.1.4   *Data distribution*

Some tests assume that the data are drawn from a normal distribution. Other *distribution-free* methods (also known as non-parametric tests) get around this assumption by converting the data into ranks or signs. In doing so, they trade off power and sometimes sacrifice confidence intervals. Where possible, we use parametric methods rather than non-parametric methods.

### 5.1.5   *What is the alternative hypothesis?*

All of the tests covered in this chapter are 'tests of equality' (other types of hypotheses, such as non-inferiority or superiority, are beyond the scope of the book). In tests of equality, the null hypothesis is that the two groups are equal (e.g., 'no change' or 'no difference' in group averages), and the alternative hypothesis is that the groups are not equal. The alternative hypothesis can be configured for one- or two-sided alternatives. This should be decided upon before running the test, not after seeing the data. One-sided tests can be appropriate but should be motivated by the prevailing understanding of the science rather than reducing sample size or lowering the threshold for statistical significance.

## 5.2   Independent samples

In this section, we detail statistical tests for two independent samples. We start with methods for interval-scaled outcomes and then methods for categorical data. In each case, we detail the data requirements, the procedure of the test, and the R function, and we finish with a worked example.

### 5.2.1 *Interval data*

As long as our data follows an approximate normal distribution, we can use either the $z$ test or the $t$ test to compare the averages in the two samples. In this section, we first show the large-sample $z$ test and then the $t$ test, which is suitable for both small and large samples.

#### 5.2.1.1 *Large sample, normally distributed data*

The $z$ test can test differences between two groups if the sample sizes are large. The term 'large' is arbitrary, but we suggest that the sample sizes in both groups be over 100.

*Data requirements*  Summary-level means, standard deviations, and the number of observations ($n$) per group, or alternatively, the data can be at the individual level.

*Assumptions*  The data are from independent groups and approximately normally distributed. The large-sample $z$ test assumes that the variances are known, which will be reasonable if the samples are large enough.

*Procedure*  We suggest using functions from the **BSDA** package. For individual-level data, use **z.test()** and for summary-level data, **zsum.test()** should be used. One sample test against a reference can be done using the **mu** argument.

```
# x and y are
# two vectors of individual level data
BSDA::z.test(
x = x,
y = y,
sigma.x = sd(x),
sigma.y = sd(y)
)
```

```
# Two sample (summary data version).
BSDA::zsum.test(
mean.x = mean(x),
mean.y = mean(y),
sigma.x = sd(x),
n.x = length(x),
sigma.y = sd(y),
n.y = length(y)
)


# One sample (summary data version).
# mu0 = test mean
BSDA::z.test(
mean.x = mean.x,
sigma.x = sd(x),
n.x = length(x),
mu = mu0
)
```

The test statistic is the difference in sample means divided by the standard error of the difference (the $z$ values). The $z$ value is compared with a standard normal distribution, and a $p$-value is calculated.

*Example 1:*   Khan *et al.* (2006) assessed the attitudes and knowledge of medical students towards medical research in a cross-sectional survey of students from a private educational institution in Karachi, Pakistan. One of the comparisons in the study was between students exposed to problem-based modes of learning (PBL) and students who received lecture-based learning (LBL). Knowledge attained was assessed with a 10-point questionnaire. The average knowledge score (SD) in 131 PBL students was 45.7 (20.9), and the average score (SD) was 55.5 (15.3) in 66 students who experienced LDL. We enter the data as follows:

```
zt <- BSDA::zsum.test(
mean.x = 45.7,
sigma.x = 20.9,
n.x = 131,
mean.y = 55.5,
sigma.y = 15.3,
n.y = 66)

zt$statistic

##             z
## -3.735877

zt$p.value

## [1] 0.0001870623

zt$conf.int

## [1] -14.941403  -4.658597
## attr(,"conf.level")
## [1] 0.95
```

The average knowledge score was 9.8 (95% confidence interval of 4.7 to 14.9) points lower in the group assigned to problem based learning than the group assigned to lecture based learning.

*Example 2:* This example compares the number of male and female live births in England and Wales. Although the data are binary and the outcomes summarised as proportions, the $z$ test can be used under the auspices of the normal approximation to the binomial. Rather than comparing the two averages directly, we compare the proportion of male live births to a reference proportion of 0.5. The null hypothesis is therefore equivalent to the proportions of male and female births being equal. In England and Wales, in 2016, there were 696271 live births, of which 357123 were males.

```
x <- 357123
n <- 696271
p <- x/n
q <- 1 - p
sd.x <- sqrt(p*q)
BSDA::zsum.test(mean.x = p,
sigma.x = sd.x,
n.x = n,
mu=0.5)

##
##  One-sample z-Test
##
## data:  Summarised x
## z = 21.549, p-value < 2.2e-16
## alternative hypothesis: true mean is not equal to 0.5
## 95 percent confidence interval:
##   0.5117340 0.5140821
## sample estimates:
## mean of x
##   0.512908
```

The percentage of live male births in 2016 was 51.3%. On the basis of $p$-value from the $z$ test we can reject the null hypothesis of equal birth rates between male and females. The reasons for this difference is not clear. See the exercises and problems section for a question using a test of proportions instead of the normal approximation.

### 5.2.1.2  *Small-sample, normally distributed data*

The $t$ test is appropriate for approximately normal, interval-scaled data. Although the $t$ test was designed for small samples, it can also be used on larger samples and with independent and non-independent (paired) groups, making it a very general approach for comparing two groups.

*Data requirements*   Individual-level data from two independent groups. The `t.test()` function will accept the data as two vectors, x and y, or a vector of outcomes *y* and a group identifier, **g**, using the formula argument y ~ **g**.

*Assumptions*   Approximate normality and independent groups. The assumption of equal variances is not required as R default to `var.equal = F` - this is Welch's test. The Welch method is more appropriate when the two groups are of unequal size. For a *t* test with equal variance assumption select `var.equal=T`.

*Procedure*   The *t*-test function returns the means in the two groups, a confidence interval for the difference (but not the point estimate of the difference), a *t* statistic, degrees of freedom (df), and a *p*-value. The standard error for the difference is not stored. The *effective* degrees of freedom in the Welch test are calculated using the Satterthwaite approximation. A generic code for running the test is given as follows:

```
# two vectors x and y
tt <- t.test(x = x, y = y)

# g is a factor indicating group membership
tt <- t.test(y ~ g, data = data)

# print all test resultss to the console
print(tt)

# estimated group means
tt$estimate

# estimated difference males (2) - females (1)
diff(tt$estimate)

# confidence interval
tt$conf.int

# effective degrees of freedom
tt$parameter
```

*Example*:  An amino acid bioactive peptide considered to be neuro-toxic in the adult brain and a potential key driver of neurodegenera-tion has been identified. Peptide concentrations from brain samples were obtained from 17 men and 21 women. The peptide concentra-tion is approximately normally distributed, so a $t$ test is suitable to test the hypothesis that there are no differences in the peptide concentrations in male and female brains.

```
data(Peptides, package = "R4HCR")

# Individual level data t test.
# Welch's test
tt <- t.test(peptide ~ sex, data = Peptides)

# estimated group means
tt$estimate

## mean in group M mean in group F
##        9.167149        8.670155

# confidence interval
tt$conf.int

## [1] 0.1292044 0.8647839
## attr(,"conf.level")
## [1] 0.95
```

The 95% confidence interval (for the difference in means) is 0.13–0.86. Thus, we are 95% confident that the true difference in peptide concentrations is between 0.13 and 0.86 units higher in men than in women.

### 5.2.1.3  *Distribution-free test for interval scale data*

In the previous example, we used a test that assumed that the data distribution was approximately normal. Although the $t$ test is robust to deviations from normality, we may sometimes want to use a method that doesn't require the assumption of normality.

*Data requirements*  As per the requirements for the $t$ test.

*Assumptions* As per the *t* test, but the assumption of approximate normality is relaxed.

*Procedure* The two-sample Wilcoxon test (also known as the Mann–Whitney test) is a rank-based method. First, the two samples are combined and assigned a rank from smallest to largest. Under the null hypothesis of no difference, the ranks would fall randomly between the two groups and the sum of their ranks expected to be equal. The ranks of one group are then summed. The expected sums of ranks under the null hypothesis are then subtracted from the observed summed ranks to form the Wilcoxon test statistic $(W)$, and the null hypothesis is rejected if $W$ is large enough. This test can be done in R using the `wilcox.test()` function. One criticism of the original Wilcoxon–Mann–Whitney rank-sum test is that it only returns a *p*-value. However, point estimates and confidence intervals associated with the rank-sum approach are available in R. The Hedges–Lehmann estimator and a distribution-free confidence interval are returned when the argument `conf.int = T` is used. The motivation for this estimator is based on how much one sample would need to be shifted to make it look like a sample from a homogenous population. In the two sample case, the estimator is the median of the differences between the two groups and not the difference of the medians as is sometimes assumed.

*Example*: We now use the Wilcoxon test on the peptide data from the previous section.

```
wt <- wilcox.test(peptide ~ sex, data = Peptides)

## Warning in wilcox.test.default(x = DATA[[1L]], y =
DATA[[2L]], ...): cannot compute exact p-value with ties

wt$statistic

##   W
## 271

wt$p.value

## [1] 0.00634413
```

```
# derivation of the Wilcoxon/Mann-Whitney statistic in R
Peptides$rank <- rank(Peptides$peptide)
xs <- with(Peptides, split(Peptides, f = sex))
f <- xs$F$rank
m <- xs$M$rank
n <- length(m)

# observed   - expected
sum(m) - ((n*(n+1))/2)

## [1] 271
```

For these data, an exact $p$-value cannot be computed (and R outputs a warning message) because there are ties in the data. The data here are relatively discrete, something which is obscured by the number of decimal places. Even though an exact $p$-value cannot be computed, a large-sample $p$-value can be calculated and used to test the null hypothesis of no difference in peptide concentrations between men and women. The small $p$-value means we should reject the null hypothesis of no difference. For these data, the $t$ test and rank-sum method lead to similar conclusions; there is strong evidence to reject the hypothesis of no difference in peptide levels between males and females. A confidence interval for the median can be found by doing the following:

```
wt2 <- wilcox.test(peptide ~ sex,
data = Peptides,
conf.int = T)
```

```
wt2$conf.int
```

The 95% confidence interval for the median difference (not shown) is between 0.18 and 0.94, which can be interpreted as that we are 95% confident the true median of the difference is between 0.18 and 0.94 units. The conclusion from the Wilcoxon test is the same as the conclusion from the $t$ test — there is strong evidence for differences in peptide concentrations between men and women.

## 5.2.2    *Binary data*

Outcomes in clinical research are frequently classified into two mutually exclusive groups (e.g., dead or alive, recovered or not). In the case of two samples, we will be interested in comparing the proportions, risks, or odds of experiencing the outcome between the two groups. The approaches to testing the differences in proportions, relative risks, and odds ratios are similar, and will often reach the same conclusion, albeit presenting the results in a different format.

### 5.2.2.1    *Large sample, all expected frequencies $>= 5$*

The following method is suitable for large-sample, binary data. The statistical test underpinning the analysis of the two-way table is the chi-square test.

*Data requirements*    Without loss of generality, we call one group the exposed group (Exposed $+$) and the other unexposed group (Exposed $-$). The outcome is either experienced (Outcome $+$) or not experienced (Outcome $-$). Thus, the total number of observations $N$ is split into four cells of a two by two table, as in Table 5.1.

*Assumptions*    The two groups (exposed positive and exposed negative) are independent. This large-sample method is appropriate if all of the expected table cell counts are greater than 5. The outcome is assumed to follow a Bernoulli trial where the outcome is either a success or a failure.

*Procedure*    There are several ways to compute measures of associations and test hypotheses for $2 \times 2$ table data. The `epi.2by2()` function from the epiR package can be used when the data is arranged

**Table 5.1.**    Layout of the data for use in the `epi.2by2()` function.

|              | Disease $+$ | Disease $-$ | Total     |
|--------------|-------------|-------------|-----------|
| Exposed $+$  | $a$         | $b$         | $a + b$   |
| Exposed $-$  | $c$         | $d$         | $c + d$   |
| Total        | $a + c$     | $b + d$     | $N$       |

**Table 5.2.** Cross-classification of aspirin use and myocardial infarction.

| Exposure | Myocardial infarction + | − | Total |
|---|---|---|---|
| Aspirin (+) | $a = 104$ | $b = 10933$ | $a + b = 11037$ |
| Placebo (−) | $c = 189$ | $d = 10845$ | $c + d = 11034$ |

as per Table 5.1. The advantage of this function is that we can choose one among the `cohort.count`, `cohort.time`, `case.control`, or `cross.sectional` designs, and the function will then calculate the appropriate measures of association.

*Example 1:* Table 5.2 comes from a five-year randomised study testing whether regular aspirin intake reduces mortality from cardiovascular disease (Agresti, 1996). We denote the exposed group as those randomised to regular aspirin use and the unexposed group as those randomised to placebo. Outcome is either experiencing (positive) or not experiencing (negative) myocardial infarction during the study period.

Of the $c + d = 11034$ assigned to the placebo arm, 189 had a heart attack in five years of follow-up. Therefore, the observed risk in the placebo arm is $189/11034 = 0.017$, or 17 per 1000. The observed risk in the aspirin arm is $104/11037 = 0.009$, or about 9 per 1000. The design is a prospective cohort, and the outcome is a count, so we select `method = "cohort.count"` to obtain a risk ratio and other measures of association with confidence intervals:

```
a <- 104
b <- 10933
c <- 189
d <- 10845

tab <- matrix(c(a,c,b,d), 2, 2)
dimnames(tab) <- list(Treat = c("Aspirin","Placebo"),
"Myocardial infarction" = c("Yes", "No")
)
```

```
rr <- epiR::epi.2by2(tab,
method="cohort.count",
units=1000)
su <- rr$massoc.detail

# the 2-way table
rr$tab[1:2,1:2]
```

```
##                   Outcome +     Outcome -
## Exposed +              104         10933
## Exposed -              189         10845
```

```
# the relative risk and 95% CI
signif(su$RR.strata.wald,2)
```

```
##      est lower upper
## 1 0.55  0.43   0.7
```

```
# p value for uncorrected chi2 test
rr$massoc.detail$chi2.strata.uncor['p.value.1s']
```

```
##        p.value.1s
## 1 2.845948e-07
```

```
# The attributable risk
signif(su$ARisk.strata.wald,2)
```

```
##      est lower upper
## 1 -7.7   -11  -4.7
```

```
# Number needed to treat
signif(su$NNT.strata.wald,2)
```

```
##      est lower upper
## 1 -130  -210   -93
```

The risk ratio (aspirin vs. placebo) is estimated at 0.55, which implies the risk of a heart attack after taking aspirin is roughly half the rate in the placebo arm. Based on these data, we can be 95% confident that the risk ratio is between 0.43 and 0.70. The very small $p$-value indicates that this difference in the number of heart attacks

**Table 5.3.** Presence of NMDAR antibodies in patients with first-episode psychosis and controls (Lennox *et al.*, 2017).

| NMDAR antibodies | Outcome | | Total |
| | Cases | Controls | |
|---|---|---|---|
| + | $a = 7$ | $b = 0$ | $a + b = 7$ |
| − | $c = 221$ | $d = 105$ | $c + d = 326$ |
| Total | 228 | 105 | $N = 333$ |

between the two groups is highly unlikely were the aspirin having no effect. Attributable risk is the difference in risks between people taking aspirin and those receiving the placebo. It can be interpreted as aspirin leading to between 5 and 11 fewer heart attacks per 1000 people. The number needed to treat is the number of patients you need to treat *on average* to prevent one additional bad outcome. In this example, it is estimated that on average, one heart attack will be prevented for every 130 (95% CI 93 to 210) patients treated with aspirin.

The `epi.2by2()` chi-square statistic and *p*-values utilise the same tests as those in the generic base R function for a two-sample test of equality of proportions – `prop.test()`. See question 1 in the Problems and exercises section of this chapter for an example where these two functions give the same chi-square statistic and *p*-value

*Example 2:*   In a study of patients aged 14–35 years, 228 with first-episode psychosis (cases) and 105 healthy (controls) were tested for the presence of N-methyl-D-aspartate receptor (NMDAR) antibodies (Lennox *et al.*, 2017). Of the 105 controls, none had NMDAR antibodies, whereas 7 of the 228 cases were positive for the antibodies (Table 5.3). An odds ratio (*p*-value) of 5.4 ($p = 0.0204$) was reported in the paper.

To analyse case-control data of this kind, we would do the following:

```
a <- 7
b <- 0
c <- 221
```

```
d <- 105

tab <- matrix(c(a,c,b,d), 2, 2)
dimnames(tab) <- list(NMDAR = c("+","-"),
"Psychosis" = c("+", "-")
)

or <- epiR::epi.2by2(tab,
method="case.control")

su <- or$massoc.detail

or$tab[1:2,1:2]

##                  Outcome +      Outcome -
## Exposed +              7               0
## Exposed -            221             105

su$OR.strata.wald

##     est lower upper
## 1 NaN   NaN   NaN
```

In this example, the OR is not defined; the `epi.2by2()` function returned NaN for the odds ratio and confidence interval. A zero in one or more of the table's cells is generally a problem for the standard method of odds ratio estimation. However, the R function `oddsratio` from the `epitools` package offers a way to work around this particular problem. By selecting `method = "small"`, the unconditional odds ratio and confidence interval are returned in place of the usual sample odds ratio.

```
# we need to reverse both columns
# and rows for the oddsratio function

or2 <- epitools::oddsratio(tab,
rev = "both", method = "small")

## Warning in chisq.test(xx, correct = correction):
Chi-squared approximation may be incorrect
```

```
# The estimated OR and 95% confidence interval
or2

## $data
##           Psychosis
## NMDAR      -    + Total
##    -     105 221   326
##    +       0   7     7
##    Total 105 228   333
##
## $measure
##        odds ratio with 95% C.I.
## NMDAR estimate      lower   upper
##     - 1.000000         NA      NA
##     + 3.310811 0.4042404  126.27
##
## $p.value
##        two-sided
## NMDAR midp.exact fisher.exact chi.square
##     -        NA           NA         NA
##     + 0.0684882    0.1026515 0.06957984
##
## $correction
## [1] FALSE
##
## attr(,"method")
## [1] "small sample-adjusted UMLE & normal approx
(Wald) CI"
```

The estimated odds ratio is 3.31 with a 95% confidence interval of 0.40–126.3. It should be noted that this approach has the disadvantage of increasing the discreteness and hence the conservatism (wider confidence intervals) of methods (Agresti and Min, 2002). For this example, it is clear that there is not enough data to draw firm conclusions about the association between the presence of antibodies and first-episode psychosis.

**Table 5.4.** Incidence of lower respiratory infections among children aged less than five years, according to their housing conditions. Data from Kirkwood and Sterne (2010).

|                      | Outcome                  |                             |                                |
| -------------------- | ------------------------ | --------------------------- | ------------------------------ |
| Housing condition    | Number of infections     | Child-years at risk         | Rate per 1000 child-years      |
| Poor                 | $a = 33$                 | $b = 355$                   | $\lambda_+ = 93.0$             |
| Good                 | $c = 24$                 | $d = 518$                   | $\lambda_- = 46.3$             |
| Total                | $a + c = 57$             | $b + d = 873$               | $\lambda = 65.3$               |

*Example 3:* This example comes from Kirkwood and Sterne (2010: p. 240). The Guatemala morbidity study enrolled 500 children aged less than five years, living in a community in rural Guatemala. The data are shown in Table 5.4.

The incidence rate of lower respiratory infection is $(24/518) \times 1000 = 46.3$ per 1000 child-years for children in good housing condition and $(33/355) \times 1000 = 93.0$ per 1000 child-years for children in poor housing condition.

```
a <- 33
b <- 355
c <- 24
d <- 518

# put into a table
tab <- matrix(c(a,c,b,d), 2, 2)

rrt <- epiR::epi.2by2(tab, method = "cohort.time")

su <- rrt$massoc.detail

su$IRR.strata.wald

##         est     lower     upper
## 1 2.006338 1.150387 3.547655
```

Analysing these data as `cohort.time` data we obtain an estimate of the incidence rate ratio. The incidence rate ratio is 2.01 with 95% confidence interval 1.15 to 3.55.

### 5.2.2.2 *Small sample, no restriction on cell counts*

If one or more of the expected cell counts is < five, Fisher's exact test can be used.

*Data requirements* As per the large sample method, but the condition of all expected frequencies $>= 5$ is relaxed.

*Procedure* Fisher's test is based on an exact distribution that can only be defined when the row and column totals are given. This test is available in R via the `fisher.test()` function. As per the other functions covered in this section, the main argument can be a two-way table in matrix form.

*Example*: This example is taken from the help page for the `fisher.test()` function, which in turn cites Agresti (1996). The example comes from R.A. Fisher, who used it to illustrate his test. Dr. Muriel Bristol, a colleague of Fisher, claimed to be able to tell whether milk or tea was added to a cup first. Fisher designed an experiment that involved Dr. Bristol trying eight cups of tea, four of which had milk added first and four had tea added first. The null hypothesis is that no association exists between the true order of pouring milk and Dr. Bristol's guesses.

```
tea <- matrix(c(3, 1, 1, 3), nrow = 2)
ft <- fisher.test(tea, alternative = "greater")

ft$p.value

## [1] 0.2428571

ft$estimate

## odds ratio
##    6.408309

ft$conf.int
```

```
## [1] 0.3135693          Inf
## attr(,"conf.level")
## [1] 0.95
```

The test provides a *p*-value and an estimate of the odds ratio. Note that this is the conditional rather than the common sample odds ratio we use routinely. It can be interpreted in the same way, and so values greater than one would be indicative of evidence against the null. The *p*-value, however, suggests that guessing 6 out of 8 cups correctly is not significant to reject the null hypothesis. Although this test was designed for experiments with fixed margin totals, such as the tea experiment, it is commonly used in designs where the margins are not fixed in advance, e.g., in observational studies.

### 5.2.3    *Categorical or nominal data*

The method for binary data easily extends to the case of more than two nominal or ordinal categories. If the data are ordinal, then the ordinality should not be ignored, as an important trend could be missed.

#### 5.2.3.1    *The 2 × k chi-square test and linear trend*

Chi-square is a test of independence between rows and columns. The linear trend test measures the degree of correlation – large values of the test statistic are evidence against independence.

*Data requirements*    Counts of successes or failures and the total number of trials for each category. For the linear trend test, an additional vector of scores is required. A score is a scale you assign to the category. In the linear trend test, the scores should reflect the order of the levels of category.

*Assumptions*    The expected table cell counts are greater than five.

*Procedure*    The `chisq.test()` function accepts a $2 \times k$ table and returns the $\chi^2$ statistics and a *p*-value corresponding to the tests of independence.

```
# where x is a 2 by k table
ct <- chisq.test(x)

# the value the chi-squared test statistic.
ct$statistic

# Degrees of freedom
ct$parameter

# expected counts under the null hypothesis.
ct$expected

# To simulate p value
ct <- chisq.test(x, simulate.p.value = TRUE)

# Test for linear trend
# x is a vector of "successes"
# n is the total number of trials
# The scores assigned to categories.

pt <- prop.test.trend(x = x, n = n, score = score)

# statistics
pt$statistic
```

*Example*: We show both methods using an example from Agresti (1996). The data are part of the R4HCR package.

```
data(Malformation, package = "R4HCR")
Malformation

##   Alcohol_consumption Absent Present Midpoints
## 1                   0  17066      48       0.0
## 2                  <1  14464      38       0.5
## 3                 1-2    788       5       1.5
## 4                 3-5    126       1       4.0
## 5                >=6     37       1       7.0
```

The Chi-square test for independence can be run in R: Despite the large sample sizes in this example, the conditions for the test (all expected cell counts $> 5$) are not met. To make this assumption, we simulate the $p$-value here rather than rely on the large-sample approximation

```
with(Malformation,
chisq.test(x = rbind(Absent,Present),
simulate.p.value = T))

##
##  Pearson's Chi-squared test with simulated p-value
##    (based on 2000 replicates)
##
## data:  rbind(Absent, Present)
## X-squared = 12.082, df = NA, p-value = 0.03598
```

This suggests some evidence against independence. We can test for a trend. The `prop.trend.test()` function allows the user to specify a score to reflect the distances between categories. The default is for equal distances. For most data, the choice of score has makes little difference, but for this example, the choice of midpoints is pivotal. The $p$-value shows evidence for a trend in infant malformation and alcohol consumption.

```
with(Malformation,
prop.trend.test(x = Present,
n = Absent + Present,
score = Midpoints)
)

##
##  Chi-squared Test for Trend in Proportions
##
## data: Present out of Absent + Present,
##  using scores: 0 0.5 1.5 4 7
## X-squared = 6.5701, df = 1, p-value = 0.01037
```

## 5.3 Non-independent samples

Non-independent (or paired) samples often originate from studies where the same group of people are measured twice, but they can also arise from matched studies. For example, in a before-and-after design, the two groups (before and after) consist of the same participants and are therefore are not independent. Appropriate methods must be used when the data come from these types of designs.

### 5.3.1 *Interval data*

#### 5.3.1.1 *Normally distributed data*

The $t$ test can be used on non-independent samples and when the data are approximately normally distributed. It is suitable for both large and small samples.

*Data requirements* A vector of differences of two measurements from the same individuals or two samples from groups that are somehow linked (e.g., with matching characteristics).

*Assumptions* Independence between groups is relaxed; in fact, it would be a grave mistake to assume independence when the groups are non-independent. Normality will hold if the measurements within each group follow an approximate normal distribution, but it may also hold even when the individual measurements do not, as the differences may be. In other words, the distribution of the differences should be checked rather than the within-group measurements.

*Procedure* The paired sample $t$ test is based on a one-sample $t$ test of the differences. The data can be supplied as two vectors, $x$ and $y$, or using the formula expression method: measurements (**y**) and group indicator (**g**) or the difference between two vectors $x - y$. When using the first two approaches, it is imperative that **paired = T** is specified in the function call.

```
# E.g.
before<-c(1.83, .50, 1.62, 2.48, 1.68)
after<-c(.878, .647, .598, 2.05, 1.06)
```

```
# data as 2 vectors
t.test(x = after, y = before, paired=TRUE)

# formula method
y <- c(before,after)
g <- c(rep("before",length(before)),
rep("after",length(after)))
t.test(y ~ g, paired = T)

# differencing method
t.test(after-before)
```

*Example 1:* Oxygen saturation (% Oxygen) was measured shortly after exercising with no face mask and, again, while wearing a cloth face mask. The same people feature in both groups, so a paired design test is appropriate. The assumption of normality is less certain, but we will assess later whether relaxing this assumption leads to different conclusions. For this analysis, we focus on the comparison between cloth face masks and no face masks.

```
data(Facemasks, package = "R4HCR")

# focus on cloth - none comparison
s1 <- subset(Facemasks,
             subset = comparison == "Cloth - None")
t.test(s1$delta)

##
##   One Sample t-test
##
## data:  s1$delta
## t = -3.4337, df = 68, p-value = 0.001018
## alternative hypothesis: true mean is not equal to 0
## 95 percent confidence interval:
##   -1.2374172 -0.3278002
## sample estimates:
##   mean of x
## -0.7826087
```

The estimated mean difference is −0.783%; therefore, on average, oxygen saturation was lower when wearing a cloth face mask compared to no face mask. Based on these data, we can be 95% confident that the true average difference is between −1.237% and −0.328%. As the confidence interval excludes 0 and the $p$-value is $< 0.05$, we can say there is strong evidence to suggest that this size difference is unlikely due to chance. The difference, although statistically significant, was not considered clinically significant as determined by a pre-specified margin of 2% (Jones *et al.*, 2023).

### 5.3.1.2 *Distribution-free method*

We now look at an approach for interval data that replaces the assumption of normality.

*Data requirements* As per Section 5.3.1.1.

*Assumptions* The assumption of approximate normality is relaxed, but this distribution-free test assumes (in strict terms) that the observations are symmetric about a common median and drawn from an *underlying* continuous population, reducing the chance of ranks being tied (Hollander *et al.*, 2014). In practice, the test is used more in settings where this isn't the case, resulting in ties. For paired data, the symmetry assumption will often be satisfied (Hollander *et al.*, 2014).

*Procedure* The Wilcoxon test is a rank-based method. The absolute values are ranked from smallest to largest. Although the ranks are based on absolute values, an additional variable is created to indicate whether the difference score was negative or positive, and the two are multiplied together to form signed ranks. For example, in the case of the before-and-after design, we would have the values like those shown in Table 5.5.

The number of positive difference scores and their magnitude contribute to the test statistic and evidence against the null hypothesis. If the intervention is associated with the outcome, then there should be a larger proportion of positive difference scores, and they will tend to have larger absolute values. If the pre- and post-measurements are not genuinely continuous and only take a limited number of integer values, then the difference scores can often be zero. In this case, these

**Table 5.5.** Example of computations involved in the Wilcoxon signed rank test.

| Pre ($X$) | Post ($Y$) | $\lvert Y - X \rvert$ | Rank ($R$) | Sign ($S$) | $R \times S$ ($RS$) |
|---|---|---|---|---|---|
| 10.8 | 10.4 | 0.3 | 2 | 0 | 0.0 |
| 13.9 | 14.2 | 0.3 | 1 | 1 | 1.0 |
| 10.6 | 15.5 | 4.9 | 4 | 1 | 4.0 |
| 7.7 | 11.3 | 3.6 | 3 | 1 | 3.0 |
| | | | | | $V = \sum RS = 8$ |

data will be excluded, which will reduce the power of the test. Ties between non-zero differences can be accommodated, but R will warn that exact $p$-values cannot be computed. If any differences (between pre- and post-measurement) are zero, they are excluded, and the sample size is reduced. However, if some of the differences share the same value, they are assigned an average rank.

```
# these are equivalent
wilcox.test(y)

wilcox.test(y[y!=0])
```

*Example*: *Face masks, continued*   We continue with the face mask example and analyse these data using the Wilcoxon rank sum test function `wilcox.test()`.

```
any(s1$delta==0)

## [1] TRUE

y <- s1$delta
wt <- wilcox.test(y[y!=0], conf.int=T)
```

```
## Warning in wilcox.test.default(y[y != 0], conf.int =
T): cannot compute exact p-value with ties
## Warning in wilcox.test.default(y[y != 0], conf.int =
T): cannot compute exact confidence interval with ties

# p value for test
wt$p.value

## [1] 0.00144591

# the estimate treatment effect
wt$estimate

## (pseudo)median
##       -1.000039

# Confidence interval for the treatment effect
wt$conf.int

## [1] -1.9999693 -0.4999804
## attr(,"conf.level")
## [1] 0.95
```

Even after removing the zeroes, a warning is still given. This indicates that we have a number of nonzero ties, which in this case is due to the rounding of saturation levels. However, the conclusions are broadly similar to those of the $t$ test, with cloth face masks being associated with a reduction in oxygen saturation compared to no mask.

### 5.3.2 *Binary data*

Similar to interval scale data, related or paired samples arise with binary data because the same subjects are assessed twice or the subjects in a study have been matched (Agresti, 2007). In this section, we look at a large-sample method, the McNemar test, and a modification to the test for small samples.

**Table 5.6.** Data specification for before-and-after design with binary data.

| Sample 1 | Sample 2 | | Total |
| --- | --- | --- | --- |
| | Success | Failure | |
| Success | $a$ | $b$ | $a + b$ |
| Failure | $c$ | $d$ | $c + d$ |
| Total | $a + c$ | $b + d$ | $a + b + c + d = N$ |

### 5.3.2.1    Large sample method

*Data requirements*    Data for this method would typically be arranged as shown in Table 5.6. Note that, although they look similar, in contrast to the table for independent samples, the rows of the table correspond to the outcome of the first measurement (sample 1), and the columns correspond to the outcome of the second measurement (sample 2). Each person contributes one observation in one cell of the table.

*Assumptions*    The only specific requirement is that the two samples have the same subjects or some other natural pairing or *dependency*.

*Procedure*    The null hypothesis for the McNemar test is that the marginal probabilities are equal $H_0 : (a+b)/N = (a+c)/N$ (marginal homogeneity). Alternative hypotheses can be one- or two-sided in nature. It can be shown that the difference between these two marginal probabilities is the same as the difference between the off-diagonal probabilities $(c/N - b/N)$; hence, the McNemar test statistic (with continuity correction) is based on the off-diagonals, $b$ and $c$:

$$t_{McNemar} = \frac{(|b - c| - 1)^2}{b + c}$$

In R, we use `mcnemar.test()` to run this test. Note that it will only return a test statistic and a *p*-value.

**Table 5.7.** The number of severe colds reported at two ages (12 and 14) for Kent schoolchildren (Bland, 1995).

|  | Severe colds at age 14 | | |
| --- | --- | --- | --- |
| Severe colds at age 12 | Yes | No | Total |
| Yes | $a = 212$ | $b = 144$ | $a + b = 356$ |
| No | $c = 256$ | $d = 707$ | $c + d = 963$ |
| Total | $a + c = 468$ | $b + d = 851$ | $N = 1319$ |

```
tab <- matrix(c(a,c,b,d),ncol=2)
mt <- mcnemar.test(tab)

# test statistic
mt$statistic

# p value
mt$p.value
```

A continuity correction is advisable when the expected values are small, i.e., less than 20 (Bland, 1995). R defaults to applying the continuity correction, but this can be switched off using the `correct = F` argument.

*Example*: The following example comes from Holland (1978) and is reproduced by Bland (1995). Respiratory symptom questionnaires for 1319 Kent schoolchildren at ages 12 and 14. Interest was in whether the symptoms' prevalence differed at the two ages. The data are shown in Table 5.7.

```
a <- 212
b <- 144
c <- 256
d <- 707

tab <- matrix(c(a,c,b,d),ncol=2)
mcnemar.test(tab)
```

```
##
##  McNemar's Chi-squared test with continuity correction
##
## data:   tab
## McNemar's chi-squared = 30.802, df = 1, p-value =
      2.857e-08
```

Alternatively, an exact version of the test can be done using the `mcnemar.exact()` function from the `exact2x2` package. This returns the results of an exact test as well as a confidence interval for the odds ratio.

```
mc1 <- mcnemar.exact(tab)
mc1$estimate
```

```
## odds ratio
##      0.5625
```

```
mc1$conf.int
```

```
## [1] 0.4553919 0.6925884
## attr(,"conf.level")
## [1] 0.95
```

```
mc1$p.value
```

```
## [1] 2.330868e-08
```

The exact test returns an odds ratio and 95% confidence interval; the odds ratio reported in the `mcnemar.exact()` test is different from the one we usually calculate $(a \times d)/(b \times c)$. Instead, it is calculated using only the off-diagonals $OR = b/c$. The fact that the odds ratio is less than 1 is consistent with fewer schoolchildren experiencing severe colds at age 12 (27%) compared to age 14 (35.4%). Something that was attributed to an epidemic of upper respiratory infections just before the second questionnaire (Bland, 1995). Extensions of the method for the binary case to multiple categories are beyond the scope of this book, and the interested reader should look to texts such as that by Agresti (2007) for methods that extend the model for matched pairs.

## 5.4 Problems and exercises

(1) Replicate the results of the comparison of risks in the aspirin trial (Section 5.2.2.1 Example 1) using the **prop.test()** function. Ensure the chi-square statistic and *p*-values exactly match those of the relative risk approach.

(2) The **esoph** dataset includes records from a case-control study of oesophageal cancer in Ille-et-Vilaine, France. The records are organised as a data.frame for 88 age/alcohol/tobacco combinations. Use **esoph** to answer the following questions:

   (a) Construct a table that has the number of cases and controls for an exposure group relating to low tobacco consumption (0–9 and 10–19 gm/day combined) and high tobacco consumption (20–29 and > 30 combined).

   (b) Use the table constructed in the previous question to estimate the exposure odds ratio and 95% confidence interval. Designate the higher level of tobacco consumption as exposure positive.

   (c) Now, use all four original groups to establish whether there is evidence for a linear trend in the risk of oesophageal cancer with increasing tobacco consumption. Assess whether the choice of scores has an impact on the conclusion.

(3) In a hypothetical study investigating the possible effects of an exposure to a carcinogen, the number of cases in the group exposed to the carcinogen was 36 over 25010 person-years, and the number of cases in the group not exposed was 18 over 20146 person-years. Estimate the incidence rate ratio and 95% confidence interval; is there evidence that exposure to the carcinogen increases the incidence rate?

(4) The following data come from a study examining the effect of aspirin on bleeding time and platelet adhesion. The variable **pre** is the bleeding time (in seconds) before the ingestion of 600 mg of aspirin and the **post** is the bleeding time (in seconds) two hours after the administration of aspirin.

```
pre <- c(10.5,19.5,7.5,4.0,4.5,2.0)
post <- c(18.5,24.5,11.0,2.5,5.5,3.5)
```

(a) Carry out a hypothesis test that a 600 mg dose of aspirin has no effect on bleeding time using a parametric test, against an alternative that aspirin increases the bleeding time.

(b) Find a distribution-free method that tests the same hypothesis.

(c) The BSDA package in R has a function, SIGN.test(), that will conduct a test based on converting the differences to signs (either positive or negative). Run the test on these data and then show that the $p$-value reported by the function is the tail-area probability of a binomial distribution with parameters $p = 0.5$ and $n = 6$.

(5) This question comes from Agresti (1996). The following data are results from a study comparing radiation therapy with surgery in treating cancer of the larynx. The outcome was whether the cancer was controlled by the treatment or not at the end of the study. Suppose the investigators were interested in whether the risk of the cancer not being controlled with radiation therapy was higher than with surgery. Using an appropriate method, calculate summary statistics and an appropriate measure of effect and 95% confidence interval to address this question. Without doing any further calculations, determine whether there would be evidence that radiation therapy is inferior to surgery.

```
dat <- matrix(c(21,15,2,3),c(2,2))
dimnames(dat) <- list(
trt = c("Surgery","Radiation"),
cancer = c("Controlled",
"Not controlled"))

dat
```

(6) The following three questions use the lung dataset from the survival package. This dataset is included in your working environment when you run the library command and does not require a data(lung) command,

(a) Carry out a large-sample $z$ test of whether the age of lung cancer diagnosis for men is the same as that for women. Is a large-sample test appropriate here?

(b) Tabulate patient sex and ECOG performance score. Then, carry out a statistical test to investigate whether they are independent, taking care to not invoke an error message from R.

(c) Carry out a test of whether there is a trend in ECOG performance by sex.

(7) The sodium content (in ppm) was measured from 20 independent serum samples:

```
sodium <- c(140, 143, 141, 137, 132, 157, 143,
149, 118, 145, 138, 144, 144, 139,
133, 159, 141, 124, 145, 139)
```

The average sodium value used to analyse serum sample is 140 ppm. (National Quality Control Scheme, Queen Elizabeth Hospital, Birmingham, referenced in Data by D.F. Andrews and A. M. Herzberg, Springer, 1985.) Carry out a test of whether the median sodium level is different from 140 ppm. Write down the assumptions underpinning the test you have chosen, and determine whether they have been met for these data.

(8) The effect of gestrinone on patients with asymptomatic endometriosis was evaluated in a randomised controlled trial (Thomas and Cooke, 1987). The primary outcome measure was a score, derived by the American Fertility Society (higher scores indicate more serious disease), given to each patient before and after administration of either a placebo or active treatment (gestrinone).

```
trt <- c(rep("placebo",17),rep("gestrinone",18))
pre <- c(1,1,1,2,2,2,2,3,3,3,3,3,5,5,6,6,6,
        1,1,1,1,1,1,1,2,2,2,2,2,3,3,3,4,5)
post <- c(0,1,2,0,0,2,3,3,5,5,5,9,1,5,4,10,12,
         0,0,0,0,0,1,1,0,0,0,0,1,2,1,2,2,1,1)
change <- post - pre
gestrinone <- data.frame(trt,pre,post,change)
```

The abstract to the original paper is as follows:

A new drug, gestrinone, was subjected to the first double blind, randomised placebo controlled trial of any treatment of endometriosis. The disease deteriorated in eight (47%) of the 17 patients prescribed placebo (95% confidence limits 23% and 71%) compared with none of the 18 patients prescribed gestrinone ($p = 0.002$). There was a difference in elimination of the endometriosis in the gestrinone group compared with placebo but this was not statistically significant ($p = 0.057$). There was a significant difference in improvement of the disease in the gestrinone group compared with placebo ($p = 0.004$), confirming that gestrinone is an effective treatment of endometriosis. Endometriosis deteriorates in at least 23% of patients; as it is impossible to predict in whom this will happen, treatment appears to be warranted in all cases.

Using the above dataset, recreate each of the numbers and confidence intervals in the abstract:

(a) ... deteriorated in eight (47%) of the 17 patients prescribed placebo (95% CI 23% and 71%);

(b) ... compared with none of the 18 patients prescribed gestrinone ($p = 0.002$);

(c) There was a difference in elimination of the endometriosis in the gestrinone group compared with placebo but this was not statistically significant ($p = 0.057$);

(d) There was a significant difference in improvement of the disease in the gestrinone group compared with placebo ($p = 0.004$), confirming that gestrinone is an effective treatment of endometriosis;

(e) Endometriosis deteriorates in at least 23% of patients.

(9) This question is from Spiegelhalter *et al.* (2004). In the statin arm of the PROSPER RCT (Shepherd *et al.*, 2002), 245 cancers occurred in 2891 patients, and 199 cancers occurred in 2913 patients allocated to placebo. Calculate the odds ratio and 95% confidence interval, and assess whether there is evidence to support a difference in cancer incidence between the two groups. Finally, work out the number of 'excess' cancers per 10000 statin prescriptions we might expect based on these data.

# Chapter 6

# Measuring the strength of association

Much of healthcare research is concerned with finding the causes and determinants of disease and morbidity. Investigation often starts by assessing the association between two variables. By associated, we mean the tendency of the value of one variable to be higher (or lower) when the values of another variable is higher (or lower). In this chapter, we consider two related methods of analysing association: correlation and linear regression. Correlation measures the degree of the association and linear regression enables the value of one variable to be predicted by the value of the other variable.

## Objectives and learning outcomes

The objectives for this chapter are to:

- introduce methods for assessing relationships between two variables
- describe methods for quantifying the strength of association between two variables
- highlight the limitations of using association to infer causality

After reading this chapter, you should be able to:

- use R to calculate correlation coefficients for different data types
- recognise the differences between linear, monotonic, and non-monotonic associations
- perform simple linear regression and predict new observations

## 6.1   Introduction

While assessing association between variables is a valuable first step in an investigation, there are some important considerations in interpreting association. First and foremost, association itself, does not justify causation. Furthermore, two variables may appear to be associated for unintended reasons. For example, (1) Sampling bias: Restricted or mixed samples can inflate the strength of association. (2) Confounding: There is a third variable which affects (causally) the two variables of interest. (3) Reverse causality: The cause and effect relationship may be in the reverse direction. The risk of sampling bias can be minimised with random sampling. Confounding can be reasonably (but not completely) avoided if we take into account confounding variables. The mechanism of causality (reversed or not) is generally difficult to establish in observational study and so analysis of association can never be used as a proof of causal effect. The following sections are some examples.

### 6.1.1   *Berkson's fallacy*

Berkson's fallacy refers to an artefactual association between two diseases/risk factors, arising from differential admission rates. Everitt (2021) gives an example of Berkson's fallacy. In an autopsy study, a lower than expected frequency of cancer among tuberculosis (TB) victims implies a protective effect of TB on cancer. However, the lower than expected frequency of both conditions occurring simultaneously could be due to the fact that people with both TB and cancer are much less likely to have been autopsied than with either condition alone, leading to a bias.

### 6.1.2   *Simpson's paradox*

Simpson's paradox is an example of confounding. A measure of association between two variables may be modified when a third variable is *accounted for*. An example of Simpson paradox is reproduced in Julious and Mullee (1994). The overall success rates of open and percutaneous surgery to remove kidney stones favoured percutaneous (78% vs. 83%). Yet, when the size of the stone was accounted for the opposite was true. When the comparison was confined to patients with small kidney stones ($< 2$ cm), the success rate of open surgery was higher than percutaneous surgery (93% vs. 83%), and when the comparison was confined to patients with larger stones ($> 2$ cm), open surgery again had a higher success rate (73% vs. 69%). This seemingly impossible result is because surgery for small kidney stones is more likely to be successful regardless of method, and percutaneous surgery is preferred to open surgery for small stones. Therefore an overall comparison of the two methods is biased because we are not comparing like with like.

### 6.1.3 *Reverse causality*

Observing an association between a potential exposure and a health outcome may lead us to suspect that the exposure causes the outcome. However, we should also consider whether the opposite could be true: the outcome is the cause of the exposure. This is what is meant by reverse causality. Sattar and Preiss (2017) argue that reverse causality may be more common than we imagine. For example, several studies have observed an association between sedentary activity or sitting time (exposure) and adverse cardiometabolic outcomes (outcome), hypothesising that sedentary activity leads to cardiometabolic disease. Whilst very plausible, a similar association would be observed if those people with cardiometabolic disease were more likely to be sedantry due to their illness than those without the disease.

## 6.2 Estimating strength of association

### 6.2.1 *Measures of association*

Association between two variables is often a linear (or straight-line) relationship, but it can also be curved (non-linear or non-monotonic). For linear and monotonic non-linear relationships we can measure the strength of association using correlation. Correlation coefficient measures the scattering of points around the underlying straight line: higher absolute value means less scattering and stronger association,

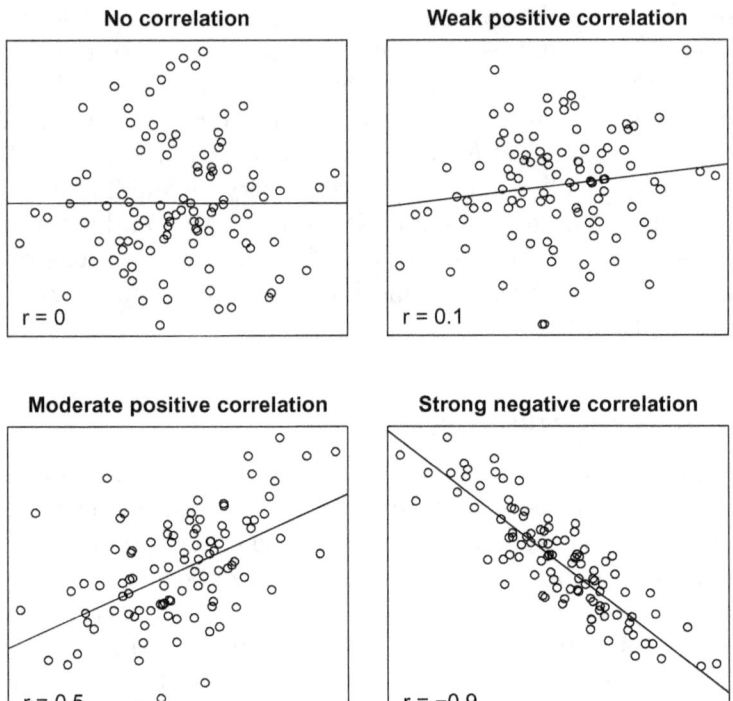

**Fig. 6.1.** Scatter plots showing different strengths of linear association with correlation coefficient values ($r$) and lines of best fit overlaid.

and lower absolute value means greater scattering and weaker association (Figure 6.1). The correlation coefficient:

- Takes value from $-1$ to $+1$.
- Is positive if higher values of one variable are associated with higher values of the other.
- Is negative if lower values of one variable are associated with higher values of the other.
- Is zero (i.e., uncorrelated) indicating there is no relationship between the values of two variables.

### 6.2.2 *Choosing the index of association*

First plot the two variables using a 2-D scatter plot and assess whether the relationship is linear. If at least approximately linear then Pearson's method is appropriate. If the relationship appears non-linear or has one or more outlying values, then Spearman's rank method is a better index to use. If non-linear and the data is not large consider Kendall's method. If the relationship changes direction (non-monotonic) then do not attempt to measure the strength using either of these methods.

### 6.2.3  *Pearson's method*

When the association appears linear and without outlying values, we can quantify the strength of a **linear** association using Pearson's product-moment correlation, which has an index commonly referred to as $r$.

#### 6.2.3.1  *Data requirements*

To calculate association we require two continuous variables of equal length. Although normality is not required for the point estimate of Pearson's $r$, the validity of hypothesis tests and confidence intervals do require normality. At least one variable should be normally distributed for tests of hypothesis, and both variables should be normally distributed for valid confidence intervals around $r$ (Altman, 1990). The two variables are assumed to have a linear association.

#### 6.2.3.2  *Procedure*

Pearson's correlation coefficient can be calculated using the `cor()` function. Incomplete or missing data can be handled using the usual `na.rm` argument. If `na.rm = TRUE`, then only the complete observations are used. A second argument, `use`, is an optional argument for specifying a method for computing covariances in the presence of missing values; readers should consult the R help pages for more details. Finally, the `method` argument allows the user to toggle between `pearson`, `kendall`, or `spearman`. These methods are covered in later sections. The hypothesis test that $X$ is not associated with $Y$ (independence) can be done using the `cor.test()` function. Confidence intervals for the correlation coefficient can be obtained using the `cor.test()` function. This requires at least four complete pairs of observations.

```
# standard method
# the default
cor(X,Y, method = "pearson")

# Confidence interval
# using formula expression
ct <- cor.test(~ X + Y,  data = data)
ct$conf.int
```

### 6.2.3.3   *Example: Ciliary beat frequency*

This example comes from Hollander *et al.* (2014) and is originally from Low *et al.* (1984). The lung's primary defence mechanism against particulate matter, viruses, and bacteria is mucociliary clearance (MCC) (Bustamante-Marin and Ostrowski, 2017). One component of MCC is ciliary activity, of which ciliary beat frequency (CBF) is an index. In a small *in vivo* study, two methods of measuring CBF, endobronchial forceps biopsy specimen and nasal brushing, were compared. A scatter plot shows a linear relationship (see Figure 6.2).

```
data(CBF, package = "R4HCR")

with(CBF, cor(Nasal, Biopsy))

## [1] 0.8659097
```

Pearson's correlation coefficient is estimated to be $r = 0.866$, which represents a strong positive association. The two different measurements of CBF are closely correlated as we might expect. The $p$-value is very small, so we can reject the null hypothesis of independence. Given the small sample size ($n = 15$), a confidence interval will be helpful. The confidence interval can be interpreted as that we are 95% confident that the true correlation is between 0.64 and 0.96.

*Testing the equality of two correlations* Suppose that we have two correlation coefficients from two independent samples and wish to test whether they are different, We can use a test based Fisher's Z transformation to assess whether the two correlation coefficients are equal. In R, this can be manually coded as follows:

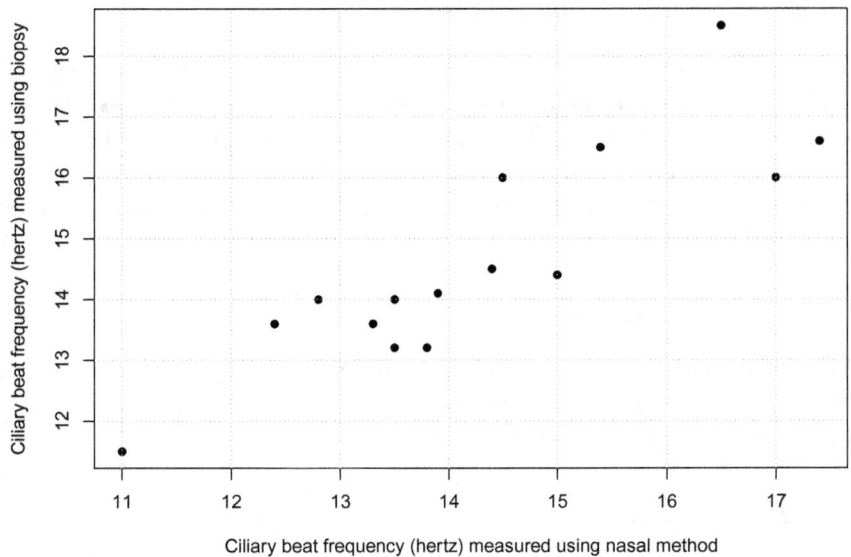

**Fig. 6.2.** Scatter plot of ciliary beat frequency measured using nasal and biopsy method.

```
## example from Kleinbaum
r1 <- 0.220
r2 <- 0.342
n1 <- n2 <- 30

# Z transform
Z1 <- 0.5*(log((1+r1)/(1-r1)))
Z2 <- 0.5*(log((1+r2)/(1-r2)))

# test statistic Z
Z <- (Z1 - Z2)/sqrt(1/(n1-3) + 1/(n2 - 3))

# two tailed p value
pnorm(abs(Z),lower.tail=F)*2

## [1] 0.6258549

# fail to reject at 5% level
```

### 6.2.4   *Spearman's rank method*

When there is a non-linear monotonic relationship, Pearson's $r$ will tend to underestimate the strength of association (as it is a measure of linear association). When the relationship is not linear, we can use a rank based method such as Spearman's rank correlation. This approach is more appropriate for non-normal or ordinal data or data with outliers.

#### 6.2.4.1   *Data requirements*

As before, two vectors of equal length representing measurement on two variables of interest. Spearman's rank correlation assumes the measurement scale is at least ordinal.

#### 6.2.4.2   *Procedure*

Spearman's rank proceeds as follows. The $X$ observations are ordered from smallest to largest and assigned a rank. This process is repeated for the $Y$ observations. Spearman's rank correlation coefficient is equivalent to the Pearson product-moment sample correlation of the ranked $X$ and $Y$ values. We use $\rho$ to denote Spearman's rank correlation. Confidence intervals for Spearman's rank correlation are not calculated with the `cor.test(...,method = "spearman")` function. This is because of the undesirable properties of the test statistic under this method (Hollander *et al.*, 2014). We know of two possible means to obtain confidence intervals in this setting. The first uses the fact that Spearman's rank correlation can be calculated using the Pearson method on the ranked values. With the Pearson method, we get a confidence interval.

```
cor.test( ~rank(X) + rank(Y),
data = data,
method = "pearson")
```

We should caution that this violates the assumption that $X$ and $Y$ are continuous and approximately normally distributed. Using the bootstrap method to obtain an approximate confidence interval is a second possibility. As with other bootstrap applications, this is not necessarily a good method for small samples but is widely applicable for large representative samples. The general form of the bootstrap method for obtaining a percentile confidence interval for Spearman's rank would be as follows:

```
# for data frame with variables X and Y
library(boot)
f1 <- function(data,i){
boot.data <- data[i,]
ct <- cor.test(~ X + Y, data = boot.data, method = "sp")
return(ct$estimate)
}
bt <- boot(data = data,f1,R = 999)
boot.ci(bt,conf=0.95,type = "perc")
```

In the presence of ties, average ranks are assigned; that is, if the two smallest values are the same, then assign one the rank of 1 and the other the rank 2. Then, assign the average $(1 + 2)/2$ to both. If there are tied $X$s and/or tied $Y$s, and **method = "Spearman"** is used, R will give a warning about inexact $p$-values – as per our example in Section 6.2.4. In this case, we can use the **pSpearman()** function from the **SuppDists** package to obtain an exact value.

```
# alternative method to calculate p value
# using SuppDists library

# q = value of the correlation
# r = number of (complete) observations

# multiply by 2 for two-sided p value
SuppDists::pSpearman(q = rho, r = n)*2
```

Hypothesis testing for Spearman's rank follows as per the previous section. We can modify the alternative hypothesis to be either that $X$ and $Y$ are negatively correlated or that $X$ and $Y$ are positively correlated. This can be done using the **cor.test(..., alternative = "less")** for negatively associated and **cor.test(..., alternative = "greater")** for positive associations.

### 6.2.4.3   Example: Five-year cancer survival

We illustrate Spearman's correlation with data on the absolute change in five-year survival and percentage change in mortality from 20 different solid tumour cancer types (Welch *et al.*, 2000).

The correlation between change in survival from cancer and mortality from cancer is estimated by doing the following:

```
data(USCancerStats, package = "R4HCR")

cor.test( ~ survival + mortality,
data = USCancerStats,
exact = F,
method = "sp")


##
## Spearman's rank correlation rho
##
## data:  survival and mortality
## S = 1437.2, p-value = 0.7355
## alternative hypothesis: true rho is not equal to 0
## sample estimates:
##         rho
## -0.08060269
```

The correlation is estimated to be $\rho = -0.08$, which suggests that a change in survival is not associated with a change in cancer mortality. We specify **exact = F** to suppress errors about computing *p*-values. The authors argued that improvements in five-year survival over time for a specific tumour might not reflect reduced disease burden and lives being saved. The original paper by Welch *et al.* (2000) provides a more detailed discussion of the trends.

### 6.2.5   Kendall's sign method

Our third measure of association can also be used for non-linear relationships. Kendall's $\tau$ is thought to have better statistical properties than Spearman's method (Kirdwood and Sterne, 2010) but computation can be slow for very large datasets. Kendall's method is based on the concordancy of pairs of ranks of data points. This is motivated by the idea that if two variables $X$ and $Y$ are associated, the order of the $Y$ values should either tend to increase with $X$ (positive association) or decrease as $X$ increases (negative correlation) — that is, they are concordant. Concordant pairs are scored +1 and discordant pairs are scored −1 and the scores are added together. An example will help explain this idea. Suppose we have two variables $X$ and $Y$ as per Table 6.1. We first rearrange the pairs of $(X, Y)$ observations so that the $X$'s are ordered from the lowest to the highest values (Table 6.2). Next we look at the ordering of the $Y$ values and score each pair of $Y$ values as +1 one if increasing, or −1 if decreasing. Starting with first and second values of $Y$ (4.0 and 7.2). As 7.2 is greater than 4.0 this is scored as +1. Next, we compare the third value of $Y$ to the first value — this is also scored +1 as 6.1 > 4.0, the fourth value of $Y$ is also higher than the first value and so is also scored +1, therefore, we have a total score of

$$(+1) + (+1) + (+1) = 3$$

Repeating this for the second $Y$ observation, we have

$$(-1) + (-1) = -2$$

**Table 6.1.** Hypothetical dataset: two variables $X$ and $Y$ measured on $n = 4$ observations.

|   | Observation number | | | |
|---|---|---|---|---|
|   | 1 | 2 | 3 | 4 |
| $X$ | 3.0 | 2.0 | 2.9 | 4.2 |
| $Y$ | 6.1 | 4.0 | 7.2 | 6.0 |

**Table 6.2.** The data from Table 6.1 rearranged so that the $X$s are ranked from smallest to largest.

|   | Observation number | | | |
|---|---|---|---|---|
|   | 2 | 3 | 1 | 4 |
| $X$ | 2.0 | 2.9 | 3.0 | 4.2 |
| $Y$ | 4.0 | 7.2 | 6.1 | 6.0 |

Note that we do not compare 7.2 with 4.0 again. The last pair is 6.1 and 6.0, which is in the 'wrong' order and so scores $-1$. In total, we have an observed score $K$ of

$$(+3) + (-2) + (-1) = 0$$

The maximum possible total score that could have been obtained is `choose(4,2)` = 6, and so Kendall's rank correlation coefficient is

$$\tau = \frac{\text{observed score } (K)}{\text{maximum possible score}} = \frac{0}{6}$$

As Kendall's $\tau$ is equal to zero, $X$ and $Y$ are not associated in this example.

#### 6.2.5.1   *Data requirements*

The data should be two vectors of equal length. Although there seems to be disagreement as to whether the data should continuous or at least ordinal for Kendall's method, the association should be monotonic as per the other methods.

#### 6.2.5.2   *Procedure*

Ties within the $X$ and/or $Y$ values are accommodated in R by adjusting the numerator to account for the ties in $X$ and $Y$ separately. For example, the following code shows an example from Siegel (1956). In these data, there are no ties in $X$, but three sets of ties in $Y$, each with two values tied.

```
# data from Siegel page 216
# status striving rank (x) and authoritarianism (y)
x <- c(3,4,2,1,8,11,10,6,7,12,5,9)
y <- c(1.5,1.5,3.5,3.5,5,6,7,8,9,10.5,10.5,12)

cor.test(x,y, method = "kendall")

## Warning in cor.test.default(x, y, method =
"kendall"): Cannot compute exact p-value with ties
```

```
##
## Kendall's rank correlation tau
##
## data:  x and y
## z = 1.7265, p-value = 0.08425
## alternative hypothesis: true tau is not equal to 0
## sample estimates:
##        tau
## 0.3877018
```

R makes a correction when there are ties in the data, as shown in the following code chunk.

```
K <- 25
Tx <- 0 # ties in X
Ty <- 3  # Ty = 0.5*sum(t(t-1)) where t = 2,2,2
N <- 12
# tau
K/(sqrt(N*(N-1)/2 - Tx) * sqrt(N*(N-1)/2-Ty))
```

```
## [1] 0.3877018
```

```
# uncorrected
K/(0.5*(N*(N-1)))
```

```
## [1] 0.3787879
```

In addition, to correct for ties in the point estimate, R also bases the *p*-value on the normal approximation to the test statistic. Hence, the output does not return a test statistic, as in the case without ties, but instead returns a *z* statistic.

Confidence intervals are not given when calling `cor.test(...,` `method="kendall")`. There are two possible solutions: one involving a large-sample approximation and another based on the bootstrap. The large-sample method requires calculating a quantity's mean and standard deviation related to the test statistic (details can be found in Hollander *et al.* (2014)). A function to do the bootstrap confidence interval function was available from the `NSM3` library at the time of writing this book (as `NSM3::kendall.ci()`). Writing your own bootstrap command is relatively easy, and the following code would provide a percentile confidence interval for Kendall's correlation coefficient:

```
# a bootstrap routine.

f <- function(data,i){
boot.data <- data[i,]
ct <- cor.test(~ + X + Y,
data = boot.data, method = "kendall")
return(ct$estimate)
}


bt <- boot::boot(data = mydata,statistic = f,R = 999)
boot::boot.ci(bt,conf=0.95,type = "perc")
```

Note that even if the original data did not have ties, each bootstrap sample will likely include ties due to the sampling with replacement. Hypothesis testing proceeds as per Pearson and Spearman. Critical values for the Kendall statistic can be obtained from the qKendall() function in the **SuppDists** package.

### 6.2.5.3   *Example: Glucose impedance*

To illustrate Kendall's rank correlation, we use data obtained by Shen *et al.* (1970) and reproduced by Hollander *et al.* (2014). The study investigated the association between the response to an oral glucose tolerance test $X$ and a measure of glucose impedance. The data come from just seven volunteers, recently released from a minimum security prison and characterised by low plasma glucose response to oral glucose.

```
data(Glucose, package = "R4HCR")

with(subset(Glucose, diabetes==0),
     cor.test(glucose, impedance,
              exact = T,
              method = "kendall")
)
```

```
##
##  Kendall's rank correlation tau
##
## data:  glucose and impedance
## T = 17, p-value = 0.06905
## alternative hypothesis: true tau is not equal to 0
## sample estimates:
##       tau
## 0.6190476
```

The correlation between glucose and impedance is estimated to 0.62 which indicates a strong positive correlation. The $p$-value (0.069) is not significant by normal standards and this probably reflects the small dataset. Note that R does not return $K$, but instead gives $T$ (a modified version of $K$).

```
# 95% confidence interval
f <- function(data,i){
boot.data <- data[i,]
ct <- cor.test(~ glucose + impedance,
data = boot.data,
exact=F,
method = "kendall")
return(ct$estimate)
}
bt <- boot::boot(data = Glucose,statistic = f,R = 999)

# Percentile confidence intervals
boot::boot.ci(bt,conf=0.95,type = "perc")
```

### 6.2.6  *Correspondence between methods*

If $X$ and $Y$ are each normally distributed, then there is a direct (mathematical) correspondence between Pearson's correlation ($r$) and both Kendall's $\tau$ and Spearman's rank correlation ($\rho$) (see Kirkwood and Sterne (2010: p. 350)). For normally distributed data, Pearson's correlation and Spearman's rank method will largely agree but Kendall's $\tau$ tends to have value that is closer to zero, unless the two variables are perfectly correlated.

### 6.2.7  *Power and efficiency*

It is easy with large sample sizes to detect weak correlations that are statistically significant but not clinically important. With smaller sample sizes we may miss clinically important associations because of a lack of power. Regardless of method and sample size, the interpretation of correlation very much depends on the context.

The distribution-free methods (Spearman and Kendall) are less efficient/powerful than Pearson's when the true distribution of $X$ and $Y$ is bivariate normal. The loss of efficiency is in the order of 10%; hence, the sample size would need to be $(1/0.9 = 1.11)$ times larger to obtain the same power as for Pearson's test. However, this will not be true when the distribution between $X$ and $Y$ is not bivariate normal, and the method of Spearman or Kendall would be preferred to Pearson's (Bhattacharyya *et al.*, 1970).

### 6.2.8  *Partial correlation*

Partial correlation measures the strength and direction of a relationship between two variables while controlling for one or more variables. Multiple linear regression could deal with many questions that could be answered with partial correlation. Although these will not entirely give precisely the same answer (as in the two-variable cases), they will tend to agree on the conclusion broadly. The **ggm** package has a function to estimate the partial correlation and to test conditional independence between two continuous variables, given other continuous variables. In practice, we tend to use regression to answer such questions.

## 6.3  Regression

Regression is a way of modelling the relationship between variables using the equation

$$y = mx + b$$

where $y$, called the outcome, response, or dependent variable and $x$ is the predictor, explanatory, or independent variable. The term 'simple' linear regression is sometimes used to describe a model with a single predictor. If there is more than one predictor, then it is called multiple regression. The values for $m$ (the slope) and $b$ (the intercept) are found by the method of least squares — the line that minimises the sum of squared differences.

Regression has two main objectives:

- It quantifies the relationship between the predictor variable and the response variable.
- It allows us to predict the response given values of the predictor.

### 6.3.1 *Data requirements*

A sample of $n$ observations from two interval scaled variables, one of which is nominated as the response variable ($y$) and one is the predictor variable ($x$).

### 6.3.2 *Assumptions*

The normal distribution assumption applies to the residuals, which is equivalent to the normal distribution for the response variable. The equal variance assumption requires that the spread (variance) of the response variable is constant for all values of predictor variable. The data are assumed to be independent. The term 'linear' refers to the fact that the response variable is a linear function of the parameters but not *necessarily* of the predictor. Hence, regression is a highly flexible technique that can model linear and non-linear relationships. All of these assumptions can be checked using graphical methods.

### 6.3.3 *Procedure*

The parameters (slope and intercept) of the model are estimated by finding parameters values that make the model fit the data best by minimizing the errors (called ordinary least squares method). In R, this is done using `lm()`.

```
lm(response ~ predictor, data = data)
```

Suppose we have data from a manufacturing process in which a glucose sensor is tested in a buffered saline solution dosed with glucose at increasing concentrations. We carry out a regression of electrical current measurements (in nA units) on glucose concentration (mmol/L).

```
glucose <- c(0,1,2,3,5,7,10,15,20,25,30)
current <- c(0.39,2.45,4.46,6.41,10.15,
13.68,18.79,27.10,35.58,45.04,56.23)
sdata <- data.frame(glucose,current)

# A regression of current on glucose.

lm1 <- lm(current ~ glucose, data = sdata)
```

The summary of the linear model is obtained using the **summary()** command, where the argument **object** is an object of **lm** class. An example follows:

```
summary(object = lm1)

##
## Call:
## lm(formula = current ~ glucose, data = sdata)
##
## Residuals:
##      Min       1Q    Median       3Q      Max
## -1.16299 -0.46210  0.07572  0.34508  1.45829
##
## Coefficients:
##               Estimate Std. Error t value Pr(>|t|)
## (Intercept)   0.68556    0.33034   2.075   0.0678 .
## glucose       1.80287    0.02266  79.565 3.96e-14 ***
## ---
## Signif. codes:  0 '***' 0.001 '**' 0.01 '*' 0.05 '.'
##    0.1 ' ' 1
##
## Residual standard error: 0.742 on 9 degrees of freedom
## Multiple R-squared:  0.9986, Adjusted R-squared:  0.9984
## F-statistic:  6331 on 1 and 9 DF,  p-value: 3.961e-14
```

The coefficients table from the regression summary have two rows: one for the intercept and one for the slope. These can be interpreted as follows. The intercept is the current (nA) when glucose concentration is zero, and the slope is the change in current (nA) for an increase of one mmol/L of glucose.

The regression summary output provides several statistics. The multiple R-squared is the square Pearson's correlation. Taking the square root of the multiple R-squared would give us the correlation between glucose and the current produced by the sensor. Two tests of hypothesis are returned in the summary output. Alongside the Coefficients estimates are standard errors for the estimates (Std. Error), *t*-statistic values (t value), and *p*-values (Pr(>|t|)). The first row, labelled (Intercept), corresponds to a test that the intercept term equals 0. Some might consider removing the intercept term from the model on the basis of the *p*-value for the intercept. This would make the regression equation

$$y = mx$$

and this model can be fitted in R by doing the following:

```
# no intercept model.
lm(response ~ predictor - 1, data = data,...)
```

We suggest that even if the test of intercept is non-significant, it shouldn't be removed unless theoretical arguments can be given *a priori* for forcing the regression line through the origin. The second hypothesis test returned on the row below (Intercept) is of more interest – the test that the slope is zero. If this null test is not rejected, then either the predictor $X$ provides little or no help in predicting the response $Y$ or it could be that the relationship between $X$ and $Y$ is not linear. If the hypothesis is rejected, we can say that $X$ is associated with $Y$ but not necessarily rule out that there is a better way to represent the relationship between $X$ and $Y$. Confidence intervals for the regression coefficients (the intercept and the slope) can be obtained in two ways. Confidence intervals (based on $t$ values) can be obtained using the confint.default() function.

```
# where obj is a linear model object
confint.default(lm1)

##                        2.5 %     97.5 %
## (Intercept) 0.03809461 1.333020
## glucose        1.75846099 1.847283
```

We usually assess the linearity assumption graphically using a scatter plot. To help assess linearity, it can be helpful to add the fitted regression line to the scatter plot. This can be done using the **abline()** function (see Figure 6.3).

The regression equation can be used to determine the mean response with a given value of the predictor on the regression line and also to predict a value of the response for a particular value of the predictor. To do both, we use the same function, **predict()**, as follows:

```
predict(lm1,newdata=list(glucose=15),
interval = "confidence")

##            fit        lwr        upr
```

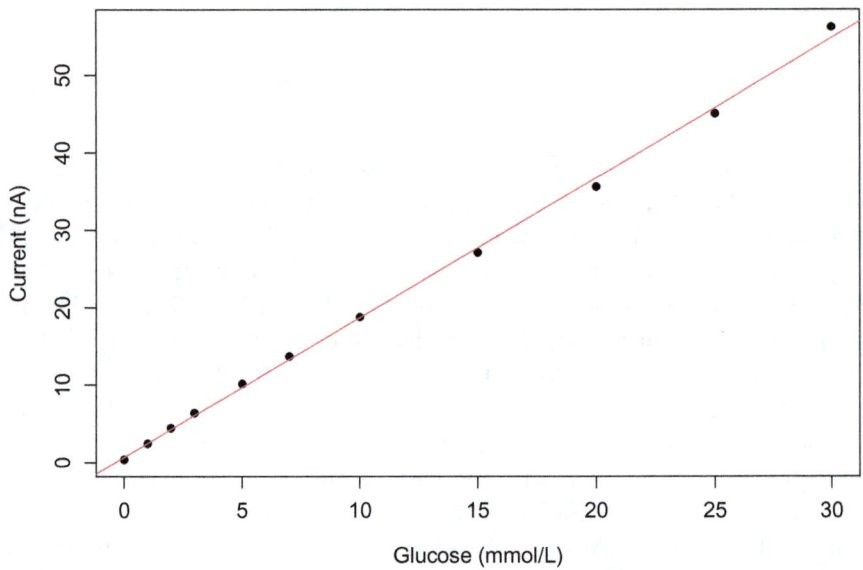

**Fig. 6.3.** Scatter plot of electric current (nA) versus glucose (mmol/L) concentration.

```
## 1 27.72863 27.17722 28.28005
```

```
# for single data point prediction
predict(lm1,newdata=list(glucose=15),
interval = "predict")
```

```
##          fit      lwr      upr
## 1 27.72863 25.96197 29.4953
```

The estimate for the mean response and for a single data point are the same, but their confidence intervals differ. The confidence interval for the mean response is narrower than for a single data point reflecting that the fact that there is more certainty around the average response than there is for a single data point.

The difference between the observed value of the response and the value predicted by the regression line is called the residual. We can access the residuals for a linear model as follows:

```
# lm1 is a regression model object from before
# first three observations
residuals(lm1)[1:3]
```

```
##          1           2           3
## -0.29555706 -0.03842886  0.16869934
```

Graphs using the residuals can be useful in assessing linearity, identifying outliers, and observing patterns in the residuals. One such plot is a plot of residuals against the fitted values (Figure 6.4):

```
# residuals vs fitted.
plot(lm1, which = 1)
```

Although there appears to be a linear relationship between glucose and current (Figure 6.3), the residuals reveals evidence of non-linearity and outlying values for high glucose values. More generally, non-linearity in the structural part of the model can also be detected in this plot if it shows a particular pattern of scattering. We can also use the residual plot to examine the constant variance assumption.

The scatter of residuals will be uniform when the variance is constant but non-uniform when the variance is not constant. For example, we may see a funneling effect in the residuals when the variance is increasing or decreasing with the value of the predictor. There is evidence of non-constant in the residuals for the glucose regression (Figure 6.4).

### 6.3.4   *Example*

Medical humanities are believed to positively impact medical education and medical practice, yet the extent of medical humanities teaching in medical schools is largely unknown. As part of a larger study, Howick *et al.* (2022) explored whether there exists a relationship between the number (mandatory or not) of medical humanities topics offered and the average world ranking in 109 accredited medical schools in the US.

```
data(MedSchools, package = "R4HCR")
m0 <- lm(Ranking ~ Humanities, data = MedSchools)
su <- summary(m0,digits = 2)
su$coefficients
```

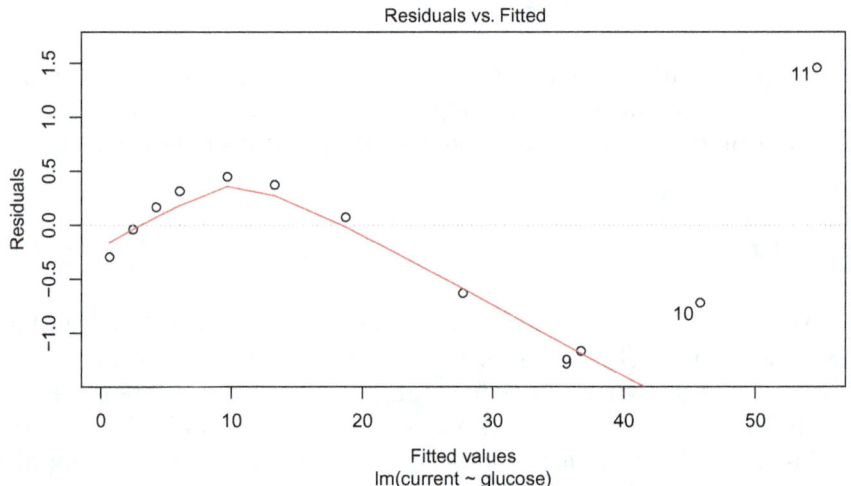

**Fig. 6.4.**   Residuals versus fitted values for the glucose sensor regression. The red line shows the smoothed trend of residual against the fitted values.

```
##             Estimate Std. Error   t value      Pr(>|t|)
## (Intercept) 274.13798  24.667099 11.113507 1.536262e-19
## Humanities  -15.98501   6.705564 -2.383843 1.889460e-02
```

Both the test of zero intercept and slope can be rejected. Contrary to what the authors anticipated, there appears to be a negative association between the number of medical humanities topics offered and the world ranking in medical schools. A residual plot from the regression indicates non-constant variance. (See the problems and exercises section for an exercise on this topic.)

## 6.4 Problems and exercises

(1) The following data represent cases and deaths from SARS-CoV-2 by age group and vaccination status. Use the data to answer the following questions.

(a) Calculate the overall case-fatality rate (deaths/cases $\times$ 10000) in vaccinated and unvaccinated groups. Calculate the ratio of the two case-fatality rates, and without doing any further analysis, determine whether the association suggests a protective or harmful effect of the vaccine.

(b) Calculate the age-specific case-fatality rate for vaccinated and unvaccinated groups. Again, calculate this ratio of case-fatalities between vaccinated and unvaccinated groups for the younger- and older-age groups.

(c) Compare your findings from part (a) with those of part (b). Try to explain, in one or two sentences, why we see what we see in such a way that a non-expert would understand.

```
cases <- c(147612,3440,25536,21472)
deaths <- c(48,205,13,389)
vaccinated <- c("No","No","Yes","Yes")
age <- c("<50",">=50","<50",">=50")
casefatality <- (deaths/cases)*10000

xtabs(cbind(deaths,cases) ~ vaccinated + age)
```

(2) The following data are taken from a larger study looking at the anatomical and pathological status of the corticospinal and somatosensory tracts and parietal lobes of patients who had had cerebral palsy. The example comes from Hollander *et al.* (2014), who cite Sylvester (1969) as the source. Run the following R code and complete the subsequent questions.

```
weight <- c(515,286,469,
410,461,436,479,198,389,262,536)
count <- c(32500,26800,11410,14850,
23640,23820,29840,21830,24650,22500,26000)
cp <- data.frame(weight,count)
```

   (a) Graph the data and assess the direction and strength of the association. Check the plot for linearity, monotonicity, and outliers.

   (b) Test the hypothesis of independence versus the alternative that brain weight and large fibre count in the medullary pyramid are correlated in subjects who have had cerebral palsy.

   (c) Show for these data that the correlation coefficient using Spearman's method is equal to the Pearson's correlation coefficient of the ranked weight and count data.

   (d) The `outliers` package performs Grubb's tests (`grubs.test()`) for one or two outliers in small samples. Use this to test the existence of an outlier in the cerebral palsy dataset. Assess the impact of excluding outliers on the correlation coefficient.

(3) These data are from a study on various psychological tests and physical characteristics of 13 dizygotic male twins from Hollander *et al.* (2014), who cite Clark, Vandenberg, and Proctor (1961) as the source. Load in the data and answer the following questions:

   (a) Calculate the strength of the linear association in the psychological test scores between twins.

   (b) Fit a simple linear regression of $y$ on $x$, and obtain an estimate of the slope of the regression lines.

   (c) Give an explanation for why the values obtained in part (a) are similar to those obtained in part (b).

(d) Find the expected score for a $y$ twin, whose $x$ twin psychological score was 210.

```
x <- c(277,169,157,139,108,213,232,229,
114,232,161,149,128)
y <- c(256,118,137,144,146,221,184,
188,97,231,114,187,230)
twins <- data.frame(x,y)
```

(4) In Section 6.3.4, it was noted that a plot of the residuals versus the fitted values from the fitted regression showed signs of non-constant variance. Plot the residuals and identify a remedy for this; check whether your solution works by repeating the residual plot with a regression line fitted with the modification.

(5) This example comes from Agresti (2007) and was first published by Hosmer and Lemeshow. The data are from a study that assessed factors associated with women's attitudes towards mammography. The women were asked, 'how likely is it that a mammography could detect a new case of breast cancer?' The responses were grouped according to whether women had never used mammography or had experienced a mammography within the past year or over one year ago.

```
experience <- c(0,0,0,1,1,1)
detection <- c(1,2,3,1,2,3)
freq <- c(13,77,144,5,28,145)
xt <- xtabs(freq~experience+detection)
dimnames(xt) <-
list(c("None","Yes"),
c("Not likely","Somewhat likely","Very
likely"))
```

(a) Calculate the percentage of women who had previous experience of mammography and who responded with 'not likely', 'Somewhat likely' and 'Very likely' when asked how likely it is that mammography could detect a new breast cancer. Comment on any trends in these data.

(b) Carry out a test of trend using **prop.trend.test**. Interpret the result.

(c) Now, calculate the correlation between the experience and attitude 'scores' weighted by the frequencies. The `cov.wgt()` function can be used to calculate weighted covariances/correlations.

(d) Finally, square the correlation coefficient calculated in the previous part, multiply this by the sum of frequency counts, and show that the chi-square statistic from the trend test is directly related to the correlation coefficient.

## Chapter 7

# Clinical measurement

Clinical measurement is the application of science and statistics to measurements on the human body, and is central to many aspects of health care. Measurements help clinicians distinguish between people with varying states of health (diagnosis), determine which patients are at higher risk of a change in health state (prognosis), or assess change over time (monitoring). Measurements should provide reliable information in order to be useful aids to clinicians. In this chapter, we examine statistical methods and techniques that can be used to evaluate clinical measurements.

### Objectives and learning outcomes

The objectives for this chapter are to:

- introduce terminology used in clinical measurement analysis
- describe methods for quantifying error in clinical measurement
- show how agreement between two or more measurement methods can be quantified
- present key features of each method and their appropriateness to specific medical applications

After reading this chapter, you should be able to:

- recognise statistical concepts of clinical measurement
- use R to summarise and evaluate clinical measurements
- interpret clinical measurement in the context of clinical problems

## 7.1   Introduction

The level of an analyte (a substance whose chemical constituents
are being identified and measured), measured in the same subject,
may yield a different result even when taken in quick succession.
Two pathologists may come to different conclusions about whether
a patient has a particular disease. A new digital device to measure blood pressure may produce a different result from the old and
trusted method used in the clinic. In each case, variation in clinical
measurement, where we may not expect it or want it, has the potential to cloud our judgement. Variations in clinical measurements are
the norm rather than the exception. When measurements on the
same person vary significantly they will be seen as less trustworthy
and not useful for guiding patient care. In contrast, when the variation is negligible or minor, they may be deemed trustworthy and
are more likely to be used for diagnosis, screening, or monitoring.
The task of the researcher, therefore, lies in quantifying the degree
of variation and its potential impact on clinical decision-making.

One way clinical measurements can vary is due to the varying
conditions under which the test is conducted. For example, blood
pressure results can depend on whether an individual is sitting or
standing, or if they are at home or in the doctor's office. Further
variations may be introduced in the analytical process, such as how
the sample is prepared or handled (e.g., transport time). Finally,
there are inherent biological sources of variation, some of which are
predictable (e.g., exercise raises serum activity of enzymes found in
muscle mass and having sex raises a man's prostate-specific antigen
level, Carobene *et al.*, 2018) while others may not. Some analytes
vary over an individual's lifetime, and many have predictable cycles
and rhythms (daily, monthly, or seasonally) (Fraser, 2013). How we
approach quantifying variation in clinical measurements will depend
on the type of measurement being studied and the context in which
it is used. Although each of the examples we show could be tackled
in several ways, we tend to prioritise certain methods over others
in particular settings. Therefore, we start by listing four methods
we have used in our research, the data requirement, and the typical
outputs from each method. These are summarised in Table 7.1.

The methods described in this section are suitable when neither measurement is assumed to be a *reference standard.* Chapter 8

**Table 7.1.** Some examples of analysis methods, data requirements, and summary measures used in the study of clinical measurement. The terms *raters* and *judges* are interchangeable and can be applied broadly, e.g., a blood test result could be either a judge or a rater.

| Objective | Data requirements | Analysis method |
|---|---|---|
| Repeatability (Section 7.2) | Two or more repeat (interval-scaled) measurements taken under the same conditions | Standard deviation of measurement error |
| Agreement (Section 7.3) | Nominal or ordinal measurements from two *raters* | Kappa analysis |
| Reliability (Section 7.4) | Interval-scaled measurements from two or more *judges* | Intra-class correlation |
| Limits of agreement (Section 7.5) | Interval-scaled measurements from two tests/devices | Bland–Altman method |

covers methods of comparing one measurement to an established reference.

### 7.1.1  *Agreement vs. correlation*

When two methods of measurement produce precisely the same result, they are said to agree. These two methods would also be perfectly correlated. However, it is not true that two perfectly correlated measurements necessarily agree. Figure 7.1 shows two hypothetical examples of measurement sets: one that agree and are perfectly correlated and another that are perfectly correlated but do not agree.

### 7.1.2  *Why test results vary*

Although there are often multiple sources of variation, the most commonly used model for interval-scaled clinical measurement assumes that observed measurements fluctuate randomly around a homeostatic set point, or 'true average'. In addition, the set points of individuals are assumed to vary around a common average. The variation in the set points of individuals is referred to as the between-subject variation, while the variation within an individual is called the within-subject variation or *measurement error*.

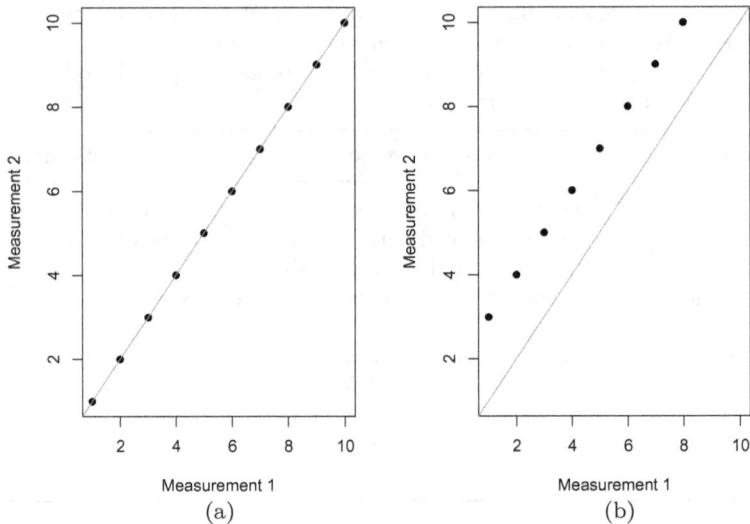

**Fig. 7.1.** Two hypothetical measurements that (a) agree and are perfectly correlated, and (b) are perfectly correlated but do not agree.

### 7.1.3 *Inter- and intra-class correlation*

When we have pairs of clinical measurements, our instinct might be to plot one against the other in a scatter plot and summarise the strength of the relationship using one of the correlation coefficients discussed in the previous chapter. However, these methods are more appropriate for measuring the strength of the association between *different* classes of data (Liljequist *et al.*, 2019) – for example, between weight and height. In other words, they are inter-class correlation coefficients. When dealing with repeated measures on individuals and, more generally, *within* a class of data, we use the intra-class correlation coefficient (ICC) to summarise the relationship. The ICC estimates the average correlation among all possible orderings of pairs and can be extended to multiple measurements, (Bland and Altman, 1996c). The ICC is the proportion of the total variation due to between subject variation. Measurements with high ICC mean it will be possible to discriminate individuals with different set points, whereas those with low values would be consistent with poor discrimination. The ICC is dimensionless, so it can be used to compare measurements of different scales.

## 7.2 Methods for quantifying measurement error

Measurement error is the variation between measurements of the same quantity on the same individual (Bland and Altman, 1996c). When the measurement error is assumed not to vary with the magnitude of measurement then we use the within-subject standard deviation (SD) as a summary measure. When the measurement error is assumed to depend on the magnitude of measurement we prefer the coefficient of variation (CV) as a summary measure.

### 7.2.1 *Indices of measurement error*

The standard deviation and coefficient of variation are the most commonly used summaries of measurement error, but other indices such as the repeatability coefficient and the reference change value are also used when communicating the impact of measurement error. We now look at these indices in more detail.

#### 7.2.1.1 *Standard deviation*

The simplest way to quantify measurement error is the SD. As the SD is expressed in the units of measurement, it can be interpreted as 'how far on average' a single test result is likely to be from the set point or *true* average for that patient. This is only useful when the measurement error is not dependent on the magnitude of the measurement.

#### 7.2.1.2 *Coefficient of variation*

When the error is proportional to the measurement's magnitude, the coefficient of variation is used to summarise measurement error. The coefficient of variation (CV) is given by the formula;

$$\mathrm{CV}(\%) = (s_w/\bar{x}) \times 100$$

where $\bar{x}$ is the sample mean, and $s_w$ the sample within-subject SD.

#### 7.2.1.3 *Measurement error coefficient*

As well as summarising the measurement error with the within-subject SD, we also find it useful to calculate $1.96\,s_w$. For 95% of single measurements, the subject's true mean or set-point will be within $1.96\,s_w$ of the observed value. For example, if $1.96\,s_w = 42$ l/min for peak expiratory flow rate (PEFR) measurement, then for 95% of measurements of PEFR, the subject's true average PEFR will be within 42 l/min of the observed value.

### 7.2.1.4  *Repeatability coefficient*

The repeatability coefficient is the maximum difference likely to occur between two repeat measurements. It is defined as $2.77\,s_w$. The difference between two measurements for the same subject is expected to be less than $2.77\,s_w$ for 95% of pairs of repeat measures. For example, if the repeatability of PEFR was estimated to be 60 l/min then we would expect the difference between two measurements on the same subject to be less than 60 l/min when their condition is stable.

### 7.2.1.5  *Reference change value*

The reference change value RCV is analogous to the repeatability coefficient for the case when variation is proportional to the magnitude of measurement. The formula for the RCV (corresponding to 95%) is 2.77 CV. The RCV can be interpreted as the value with which 95% of differences (from the first measurement) will be less than, for the same patient under stable conditions. Note that the interpretation is in terms of percentages rather than in terms of absolute changes (Fraser, 2013). Suppose the CV for serum cholesterol concentration is 6.21%, then the RCV is $2.77 \times 6.21 = 17.2\%$, and we would expect 95% of differences to be less than 17.2% of the first serum cholesterol value. For example, for two measurements on the same person of 6.60 mmol/L and 5.82 mmol/L, the change is 12% and less than the RCV value. We would have no evidence that the true serum cholesterol has changed.

## 7.2.2  *Measurement error independent of the magnitude of measurement*

The assumption of measurement error independent of the magnitude of measurement will not be appropriate for all biochemical tests used in clinical practice, but it is the simplest approach and thus represents a natural starting point.

### 7.2.2.1 *Data requirements*

At a minimum, there should be at least two measurements or *ratings* per person, taken under identical (or similar) condition(s).

### 7.2.2.2 *Assumptions*

The measurements should be continuous, and the differences following a normal distribution.

### 7.2.2.3 *Procedures*

The measurement error in this model is estimated using the within-person SD ($s_w$). This can be done by taking either the square root of the average of the within-person variances or from an ANOVA analysis. The direct method is the simplest, but the ANOVA method has the advantage of also calculating the between-subject variation. The two methods will agree when each subject has the same number of repeated measurements. Before proceeding with the estimation, we should check that the measurement error does not depend on the magnitude of the measurement. We can do this with a simple scatter plot of the variation in repeated measurements (for a particular individual) and the average within-subject measurements. Associations can be checked visually and quantified with a correlation coefficient.

```
# Assuming dt is a matrix/data frame where each
# row represents a patient and the columns represent
# sample number from 1,2,...,K, labeled y1,y2,y3

# estimate of measurement error using direct method
# first step calculates variance by row
rowVars <- apply(dt,1,var)
avgVar <- mean(rowVars)
sqrt(avgVar)

# ANOVA Method
av <- anova(lm(y ~ as.factor(subject), data = dt))
var.within <- av$`Mean Sq`[2]

# measurement error
sqrt(av$`Mean Sq`[2])
```

### 7.2.2.4   *Example: Peak expiratory flow rate*

We use data from Bland and Altman (1996b) on repeated peak expiratory flow rate (PEFR) measurements for 20 schoolchildren. It has columns representing the repeat PEFR measurements for 20 children, the within-subject mean, and the within-subject SD.

```
data(PEFR,package = "R4HCR")

# check to see if error is proportional to the mean
ct <- with(PEFR, cor.test(mean, sd))
ct$p.value

## [1] 0.667981
```

There is very little evidence to suggest an association between the within-subject SD and mean PEFR values, so we proceed with estimating the common SD. Here, we use the ANOVA method, which first requires reshaping the data from a wide format into a long format.

```
PEFR_long <- reshape(PEFR,
direction = "long",
varying = list(names(PEFR)[2:5]),
v.names = "PEFR",
idvar = "subject",
drop = c("mean","sd"))

av <- anova(lm(PEFR ~ as.factor(subject),
data = PEFR_long))
var.within <- av$`Mean Sq`[2]

# within-subject standard deviation in l/min
sw <- sqrt(av$`Mean Sq`[2])
round(sw,3)

## [1] 21.46

# same as
sqrt(mean(apply(PEFR[,2:5],1,var)))

## [1] 21.45975
```

```
# measurement error interval
c(-1,1)*1.96 * sw
```

```
## [1] -42.06111  42.06111
```

```
# Measurement error coefficient
1.96 * sw
```

```
## [1] 42.06111
```

```
# repeatability coefficient
2.77 * sw
```

```
## [1] 59.44351
```

The within-subject standard deviation is estimated to be 21.5 l/min. On average, we would expect the observed measurements to be 21.5 l/min away from an individual's 'true' PEFR (for any set-point value) and for 95% of measurements, the true PEFR to be within 42 l/min of the observed. The repeatability coefficient is estimated to be 59.5 l/min, and so the difference between two measurements on the same individual will not be more than 59.5 l/min for 95% of pairs of observations. If the difference between two consecutive PEFR measurements was larger than this, we would interpret it as evidence of a change in the patient's underlying condition.

## 7.2.3 *Measurement error proportional to the magnitude of measurement*

If the within-subject SD of a measurement is proportional to the magnitude of the measurement, then a common within-subject SD would not be appropriate. If measurement error increases with the magnitude of measurement, then a common value would be too large for lower values of the test and too small for higher values of the test. In this case, we need an approach that allows the measurement error to increase with the magnitude of the measurement.

### 7.2.3.1 *Data requirements*

The requirements are as per the previous method (see Section 7.2.2.1).

### 7.2.3.2   Assumptions

This method is suitable if the differences tend to increase or decrease as the magnitude of measurement increases. This can be checked by plotting the average of measurements against the differences.

### 7.2.3.3   Procedure

The following method is based on log transformations of the test values. Log transformations are a general method for minimising the dependency between the variance and the magnitude of measurement. It doesn't matter which base of logarithm you choose, but the base used for transforming should be the same as that used when back-transforming. We give the generic code in the following for log base $e$ (natural logarithm) and log base 10.

Once the data are log-transformed, we can apply the same calculations as before to the log-transformed data and then back-transform to obtain the results in their original units. This method of transformation leads to some notable differences from the previous method. The first is that the back-transformed within-person SD is a *geometric* within-subject SD. Provided that this SD is not large compared to the magnitude of the measurement, the geometric within-person SD is approximately equal to the CV (Bland and Altman, 1996a). Therefore, we default to using the CV as a summary measure of measurement error when the error is proportional to the mean. Secondly, although the measurement error interval is symmetric about the true value or *set point* on the log scale, once back-transformed, it is asymmetric. The CV can be calculated from the within-subject SD on the log scale by doing the following:

```
# Approx coefficient of variation (%)
(exp(log_sw) - 1)*100
```

### 7.2.3.4   Example: Duplicate salivary cotinine measurements

To illustrate the method when the measurement error is proportional to the mean, we use data from Bland and Altman (1996a). The data consist of duplicate salivary cotinine measurements for a group of Scottish schoolchildren. First, we plot the absolute differences between repeat cotinine measurements (range) against the mean

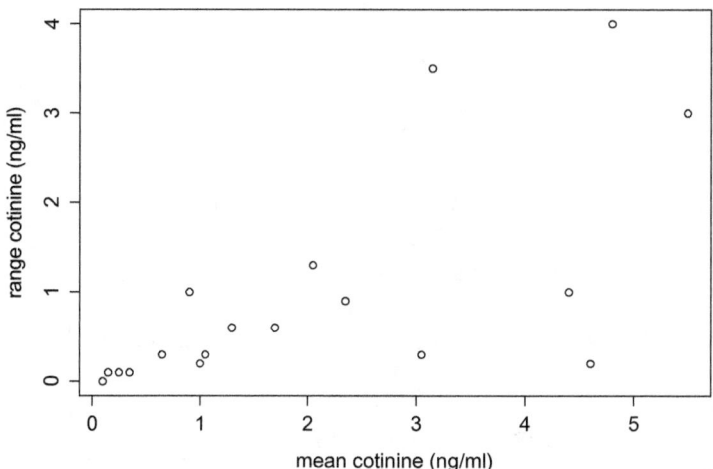

**Fig. 7.2.** Range of differences in repeat salivary cotinine measurements (*y*-axis) against mean salivary cotinine (*x*-axis) for 20 schoolchildren.

of the two repeat cotinine measurements for each child, and assess whether there is any evidence of a trend for the differences to increase with the magnitude of measurement. We then calculate the correlation between the mean and the range.

Figure 7.2 shows a strong positive association between mean cotinine and the differences in repeat cotinine measurements. After log transformation, the correlation is reduced significantly.

```
# load in data
data(Cotinine, package = "R4HCR")

# this log transforms the data
Cotinine$log10cot1 <- log10(Cotinine$cotinine1)
Cotinine$log10cot2 <- log10(Cotinine$cotinine2)
logmean <- rowMeans(cbind(Cotinine[,c(4,5)]))
logrange <- abs(Cotinine[,4] - Cotinine[,5])
```

In the original paper, Bland and Altman used `log10`, but the same *end* effect can be achieved using any other base. Now, we are satisfied that the association has been minimised, and we can proceed as before.

```
Cotinine_long <- reshape(Cotinine, direction = "long",
varying = list(names(Cotinine)[4:5]),
v.names = "cotinine",
idvar = "subject")

av <- anova(lm(cotinine ~ as.factor(subject),
              data = Cotinine_long))
var.within <- av$`Mean Sq`[2]
```

The within-subject SD on the log scale is estimated as follows.

```
# within-subject standard deviation on log scale
log_sw <- sqrt(av$`Mean Sq`[2])
round(log_sw,3)
```

```
## [1] 0.175
```

We now calculate the repeatability coefficient on the log scale and the CV and RCV.

```
# Measurement error coefficient (on log scale)
1.96 * log_sw
```

```
## [1] 0.3423413
```

```
# back-transformed measurement error coefficient
10^(1.96 * log_sw)
```

```
## [1] 2.199588
```

```
# Approx coefficient of variation (%)
(10^(log_sw)-1)*100
```

```
## [1] 49.50782
```

```
# RCV
2.77 * 49.5
```

```
## [1] 137.115
```

The back-transformed measurement error coefficient is 2.2. We can interpret this value in the following way. Suppose a child's cotinine measurement is 2.7 ng/ml, then the child's true values probably lies somewhere between $2.7/2.2 = 1.22$ ng/ml and $2.7 \times 2.2 = 5.94$ ng/ml. The CV is estimated to be 49.5% and the RCV is 137%. The estimate of within-subject variability for cotinine is very large, and too large for the approximation of CV and RCV to be reliable. In general, this approximation will be appropriate provided the standard deviation is not large compared with the level of measurement Bland and Altman (1996a).

## 7.3 Agreement between nominal or ordinal measurements

When our clinical measurements are nominal (e.g., 'yes' or 'no') or ordinal, we can use kappa analysis to measure how often two or more raters or judges agree. Some controversy surrounds the utility of kappa because its value can depend on the marginal distributions (Agresti, 1996). For example, suppose two radiologists were asked to rate 100 images to determine the presence or absence of a condition (Table 7.2). How should we summarise the agreement of the two radiologists? We could summarise as an overall percentage agreement. That would be $(38 + 45)/100 = 83\%$ for these data. The problem with this simple approach is that 1) it does not take into account where the agreement is in the table, and 2) it does not consider the chance agreement between two radiologists even if they were just guessing. The expected frequency under the null hypothesis of no association can be calculated (Table 7.3). Thus the expected agreement just by chance is $21.6 + 28.6 = 50.2$, which is 50.2% of

**Table 7.2.** Cross-tabulated results of two hypothetical radiologists rating 100 images as either present or absent for some condition.

| | | First radiologist | | |
| --- | --- | --- | --- | --- |
| | | Present | Absent | Total |
| Second radiologist | Present | 38 | 10 | 48 |
| | Absent | 7 | 45 | 52 |
| | Total | 45 | 55 | 100 |

**Table 7.3.**   Expected frequency by chance corresponding to Table 7.2.

|                    |         | First radiologist |                       |
|                    |         | Present           | Absent                |
|--------------------|---------|-------------------|-----------------------|
| Second radiologist | Present | $48 \times 45/100 = 21.6$ | $48 \times 55/100 = 26.4$ |
|                    | Absent  | $52 \times 45/100 = 23.4$ | $52 \times 55/100 = 28.6$ |

the total. So, how much better than 0.502 were the radiologists? We can express this in terms of the proportion of maximum agreement. That is, $(0.83 - 0.50)/(1 - 0.50) = 0.66$.

This measure of agreement is called kappa. It has a maximum value of 1 when the agreement is perfect, 0 for no agreement better than by chance. If kappa is negative, it indicates worse than chance agreement. The kappa statistic is defined as;

$$\kappa = \frac{\text{observed agreement} - \text{chance agreement}}{1 - \text{chance agreement}}$$

The kappa value can be interpreted as follows: values equal to 0 correspond to agreement no better than chance; values in the ranges 0.01–0.20, 0.21–0.40, 0.41–0.60, and 0.61–0.80 indicate slight, fair, moderate, and substantial agreement, respectively. Kappa values in the range 0.81–1 indicate almost perfect agreement. The agreement between the radiologists in Table 7.2 shows substantial agreement as the kappa is 0.66. Although we can say there is substantial agreement between two radiologists, it would be more meaningful to inspect the table of frequencies as many different tables will have similar kappa. The degree of acceptable agreement should be judged on the grounds of clinical context.

The kappa statistic can be influenced by the prevalence (the distribution of categories) and bias (the systematic differences in how raters classify). Low prevalence can give an artificially low kappa values and high prevalence settings tend to inflate the kappa statistic. The presence of bias between raters tends to lead to artificially low estimates of agreement using kappa. For these reasons, a prevalence and bias corrected kappa value (PABAK) may be helpful when interpreting agreement in these situations.

### 7.3.1  *Data requirements*

Two judges rate each patient into one of $k$ categories. The judges ratings can be either nominal (e.g., absent or present) or ordinal (e.g., low, medium, high). The data can be patient level with each row pertaining to a single patient and the rating of two judges. The data can also be summarised in a $k$ by $k$ table.

### 7.3.2  *Assumptions*

There are two assumptions made about independence. The first is that patients or subjects are independent (they only feature once in the data), and the second is that the judges ratings are independent (they do not confer) (Sim and Wright, 2005).

### 7.3.3  *Procedure*

For PABAK analysis, the `epi.kappa()` function from the `epiR` package can be used. For weighted kappa, we use the `Kappa()` function from the `vcd` package. Both will test hypotheses and calculate confidence intervals.

```
# epiR where tab is a 2 * 2 table.
epiR::epi.kappa(tab)

# for linear weights.
vcd::Kappa(tab,weights = "Equal-Spacing")

# for quadratic weights.
vcd::Kappa(tab,weights = "Fleiss-Cohen")
```

In contrast to the usual kappa (unweighted) which does not take into the magnitude of disagreement between raters, the weighted kappa penalises differences of greater magnitude more than smaller differences (Sim and Wright, 2005). Different methods of weighting are available, including linear and quadratic weights, and will produce different values of kappa. Suppose a weighted kappa is applied to a nominal scale with four categories. With linear weights, differences of one on the nominal scale would be weighted as 2/3, differences of two as 1/3, and differences of three as 0. With quadratic weights, differences of one are given a higher weight than those given in the linear method at 0.89, as would the differences of two at 0.56. Differences of three are weighted as 0 with both linear and quadratic weights. With unweighted kappa, exact agreements are weighted as one, while all disagreements are weighted as 0.

### 7.3.4  *Example*

The PTX dataset is synthesised from a multicentre, blinded, fully crossed, multi-case, multi-reader study conducted between October 2021 and January 2022. Readers in the study rated plain chest X-ray images and scored one if they thought a pneumothorax was visible and zero otherwise. In addition, they gave their degree of confidence on a four-point Likert scale. The raters were blinded to each other's ratings.

```
data(PTX, package = "R4HCR")

# 2-way table
(tab <- with(PTX, table(PTX1,PTX2)))

##        PTX2
## PTX1   0    1
##     0 139  22
##     1  20  19

# Kappa analysis from a table.
k1 <- epiR::epi.kappa(tab)

# prevalence index
k1$pindex


##    est          se       lower      upper
## 1 0.6 0.03859728 0.5243507 0.6756493
```

```
# bias index
k1$bindex
```

```
##    est          se        lower        upper
## 1 0.01 0.03999687 -0.06839243 0.08839243
```

```
# Kappa
k1$kappa
```

```
##          est         se      lower      upper
## 1 0.3438525 0.07067615 0.2053298 0.4823752
```

```
# prevalence- and bias-adjusted kappa
k1$pabak
```

```
##   est     lower      upper
## 1 0.58 0.4538626 0.6885205
```

```
# Agreement of confidence measured on 4-point Likert
  scale
tab2 <- with(PTX, table(Conf1,Conf2))
vcd::Kappa(tab2,weights = "Equal-Spacing")
```

```
##              value    ASE     z Pr(>|z|)
## Unweighted 0.1286 0.04913 2.617 0.008867
## Weighted   0.1495 0.05065 2.951 0.003170
```

```
# quadratic weights
vcd::Kappa(tab2, weights = "Fleiss-Cohen")
```

```
##              value    ASE     z Pr(>|z|)
## Unweighted 0.1286 0.04913 2.617 0.008867
## Weighted   0.1794 0.06373 2.815 0.004874
```

The agreement between the two readers on whether a pneumothorax is present or absent is only fair but higher than what we would expect by chance (as indicated by the confidence interval). The bias index is low, but the prevalence index is high; therefore, the PABAK estimate is higher than the standard unadjusted kappa statistic.

The analysis of 4-point Likert scale confidence scores shows slight agreement (kappa = 0.13) using unweighted kappa. The effect of applying linear or quadratic weights increases the agreement but the difference is negligible. However, we should consider weighting whenever there are more than 2 categories.

## 7.4 Agreement with interval-scaled data

In the previous section, we discussed methods for quantifying measurement error in repeated interval scaled data. We then looked at quantifying agreement when the measurement was nominal or ordinal. We now discuss a method for quantifying agreement when the measurement is interval scaled, the interclass correlation coefficient (ICC). The ICC summarises the degree of variation between subjects relative to the total variation (the sum of the between-subject and within-subject variation). When the within-subject variation is small relative to the total variation, the measurements will be closely correlated, and hence the ICC will be high. When the within-subject variation is large relative to the total variation, measurement will not be closely correlated and the ICC will be lower.

### 7.4.1 Data requirements

A sample of $n$ targets (or individuals) is rated independently by $k$ judges or *tests* in the form of an $n \times k$ matrix or `data.frame`. The ratings are assumed to be interval-scaled measurements. Table 7.4

**Table 7.4.** A hypothetical study with $n = 4$ targets rated by $k = 4$ judges in a fully crossed design.

| Target | Judge | | | |
|--------|-------|---|---|---|
|        | 1     | 2 | 3 | 4 |
| 1      | 2     | 3 | 4 | 6 |
| 2      | 5     | 6 | 7 | 9 |
| 3      | 0     | 1 | 2 | 4 |
| 4      | 3     | 4 | 5 | 7 |

shows a simple example of such a design. The term judge refers to any one person or method of measurement. For example, judges could refer to two cardiologists using an echocardiographic unit to measure left ventrilcle filling pressure, but judges could also refer to different devices measuring peak expiratory flow rate (PEFR) (Müller and Büttner, 1994).

### 7.4.2  *Assumptions*

The ICC statistics are estimated using ANOVA and so share the same assumptions: normality, constant variance, and no systematic change from the first measurement to the second or third readings.

### 7.4.3  *Procedure*

Although there are other packages, we suggest using the `icc()` function from the `irr` package. This package calculates ICC statistics for one- and two-way models, and single or average units of analysis. Confidence intervals for the ICC are also given. Before running the analysis, we should consider the following three options.

#### 7.4.3.1  *Unit of analysis*

The (first and perhaps simplest) consideration is whether the unit of analysis should be a single measurement or the average. We believe that, unless there is a clinical justification to do so otherwise, the analysis should be based on a single measurement. Here, the single measurement refers to a single measurement from each judge and the average implies averaging over the measurements in the study. The average method will always have an ICC that is equal to or greater than the single-unit ICC and therefore should only be used when it is appropriate.

#### 7.4.3.2  *Agreement or consistency*

The `icc()` function calculates agreement or consistency. The choice depends on the research question. Choose the 'agreement' option if the interest is about whether judges assign the same scores in the measurement scale. Choose the 'consistency' option if the interest is relative ranking order of targets given by each judge. In other words, agreement ICC quantifies the absolute agreement and consistency ICC quantifies correlation of rank-order (McGraw and Wong, 1996).

For example, Table 7.5 shows the data from before but with raw scores replaced by their ranks. We see that the judges give the same relative ranking, so they are perfectly consistent.

### 7.4.3.3 *One-way or two-way model*

Finally, we consider the option of a one-way or two-way model. A one-way model should only be selected if the design of the study means that each target is rated by a different set of judges, i.e., the design is not fully crossed. Table 7.6 shows a hypothetical example of such a design.

With this design, the variations due to judges, the interactions between judges and targets, and random errors are not separable

**Table 7.5.** The data from Table 7.4 but with the raw scores replaced by their ranks.

| Target | Judge 1 | 2 | 3 | 4 |
|--------|---------|---|---|---|
| 1 | 2 | 2 | 2 | 2 |
| 2 | 4 | 4 | 4 | 4 |
| 3 | 1 | 1 | 1 | 1 |
| 4 | 3 | 3 | 3 | 3 |

**Table 7.6.** Hypothetical layout of a non-fully crossed design in which *not every* judge rates each target. The letter Y means the target has been rated, and a dot means the target has not been rated by that judge.

| Target | Judge A | B | C | D | E | F |
|--------|---------|---|---|---|---|---|
| 1 | Y | Y | . | . | . | . |
| 2 | . | . | Y | Y | . | . |
| 3 | . | . | . | . | Y | Y |

(Shrout and Fleiss, 1979). In our experience, this design is less common than one in which each judge rates each target (fully crossed design). With a fully crossed design, as the same $k$ judges rate all $n$ targets, the two-way table is appropriate. The notation used in the R function we recommend is different from that used in a highly cited paper on ICC (Shrout and Fleiss, 1979). In that paper, the authors describe six different versions of the ICC statistic and label these according to the study design and unit of analysis. We believe it is easier to select the ICC according to the three criteria we have already mentioned: (1) the unit of analysis, (2) agreement or consistency, and (3) one-way or two-way model. However, one must recognise that others may look to replicate the approach adopted by Shrout and Fleiss (1979). We now show how the two approaches can be reconciled.

```
# Notation and models used in
# Shrout and Fleiss

# arguments shortened here are
# one = oneway
# two = twoway
# agree = agreement
# consist = consistency

# ICC(1,1)
irr::icc(ratings,model = "one",
        type = "agree",unit = "single")

# ICC(2,1)
irr::icc(ratings, model = "two",
        type = "agree",unit = "single")

# ICC(3,1)
irr::icc(ratings,model = "two",
        type = "consist",unit = "single")
```

```
# ICC(1,k)
irr::icc(ratings,model = "one",
        type = "agree",unit = "average")

# ICC(2,k)
irr::icc(ratings,model = "two",
        type = "agree",unit = "average")

# ICC(3,k)
irr::icc(ratings,model = "two",
        type = "consist",unit = "average")
```

### 7.4.4   Example

These data are from Müller and Büttner (1994). Two observers measured cardiac output in 23 patients using Doppler echocardiography. The unit of analysis is 'single' because, in practice, echocardiography would be performed only once. The design is fully crossed, as both judges rate all 23 targets. Finally, we calculate the agreement and consistency ICCs, which are equivalent to ICC(2,1) and ICC(3,1) used by Shrout and Fleiss (1979).

```
data(Doppler, package = "R4HCR")

irr::icc(Doppler,
model = "twoway",
type = "agreement",
unit = "single")

##  Single Score Intraclass Correlation
##
##     Model: twoway
##     Type : agreement
##
##     Subjects = 23
##       Raters = 2
```

```
##    ICC(A,1) = 0.753
##
## F-Test, H0: r0 = 0 ; H1: r0 > 0
## F(22,1.98) = 23.5 , p = 0.0429
##
## 95%-Confidence Interval for ICC Population Values:
##   -0.061 < ICC < 0.933
```

The agreement ICC is estimated at 0.75, with a 95% confidence interval −0.06 to 0.93. The very wide confidence interval (which includes negative values) reflects the small sample size in this example. The consistency ICC (not shown) is much higher, at 0.918, and indicates that although the two judges are only in moderate absolute agreement, they are consistent in ranking the targets.

## 7.5   Limits of agreement of interval-scaled data

Before a new measurement method or device can be used in place of an established method, we will often need to demonstrate agreement between the new and old measurements. The most common analysis for this type of comparison is called Bland-Altman analysis. This method principally works by finding the limits of agreement between a new and old measurement method.

Here, we use the language of 'new' and 'old' (method), but this should not limit the generality of this method.

### 7.5.1   *Method for uniform differences*

By 'uniform', we mean that the mean and standard deviation of the differences do not depend on the scale of measurement. This should be the starting assumption for any Bland–Altman analysis, but it may not always be the case. Later sections will relax the assumption of uniform differences.

### 7.5.1.1  Data requirements

The data should be paired at the individual patient level, with each subjects measured (simultaneously) on 2 devices or systems of measurement.

### 7.5.1.2  Assumptions

We assume that the differences are normally distributed and uniform with respect to the average measurement. This is equivalent to the constant variance assumption.

### 7.5.1.3  Procedure

First, calculate the differences, $d = \text{new} - \text{old}$, and the average of the two measurements, $a = (\text{new} + \text{old})/2$. Next, take the bias as the average of d ($\bar{d}$), and also calculate the standard deviation of $d$ ($s_d$). Finally, the 95% limits of agreement are;

$$\bar{d} \pm 1.96 \times s_d \qquad (7.1)$$

The limits of agreement represent a range within which 95% of the differences in measurements between two methods are expected to lie.

Confidence intervals for the bias and the limits of agreement can also be calculated. These are based on a $t$-distribution. It is common to plot the differences on the $y$-axis and averages on the $x$-axis, with lines for the bias and limits of agreement – this is often referred to as a Bland–Altman plot.

### 7.5.1.4  Example: Systolic blood pressure

We use data from Bland and Altman (1999). Systolic blood pressure measurements were made simultaneously by two observers (J and R) and an automatic blood pressure measuring machine (S). The data are available from the R4HCR package. We first plot the data for one of the observers against the machine measurement in a standard scatter plot (Figure 7.3).

```
with(Systolic,
plot(J1,S1,
xlab = "Systolic BP, observer J (mm Hg)",
ylab = "Systolic BP, machine S (mm Hg)")
)
abline(a = 0 , b = 1)
```

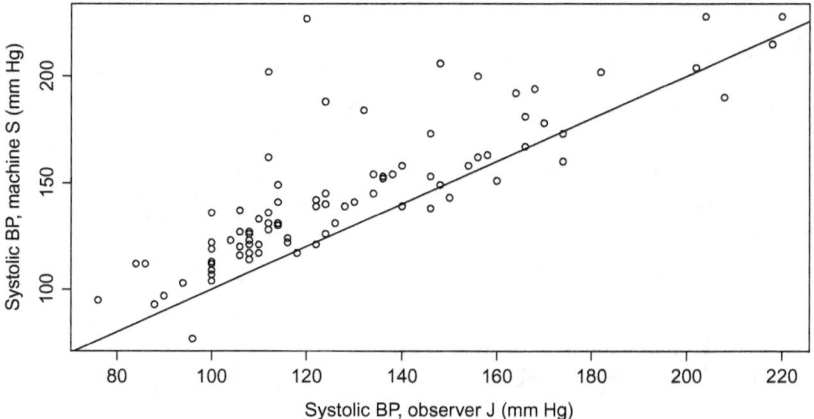

**Fig. 7.3.** Systolic blood pressure (mmHg) as measured by observer J against an automatic machine.

It is clear from this plot that the machine tends to read higher. We now show how to perform the Bland Altman analysis for these data.

```
data(Systolic, package = "R4HCR")
# differences (S1 = machine, J1 = observer)
d <- with(Systolic, S1 - J1)
a <- with(Systolic, (S1 + J1)/2)
n <- length(d)
zalpha <- 1 - 0.05/2 # for 95% limits of agreement

# bias
(bias <- mean(d))
```

```
## [1] 16.29412
```

```
# standard deviation of differences
# sd(d)
# lower and upper limit of agreement (95%)
(low.loa <- bias - qnorm(zalpha)*sd(d))
```

```
## [1] -22.14272
```

```
(up.loa <- bias + qnorm(zalpha)*sd(d))
```

```
## [1] 54.73096
```

```
# variance/std error of limits of agreement
var.loa <- sd(d)^2/n + qnorm(zalpha)^2*(sd(d)^2/
  (2*(n-1)))
se.loa <- sqrt(var.loa)
```

```
# confidence interval for the bias
bias + c(-1,1)*qt(zalpha,n-1)*(sd(d)/sqrt(n))
```

```
## [1] 12.06412 20.52411
```

```
# confidence intervals for lower limit of agreement
low.loa - qt(zalpha,n-1)*se.loa
```

```
## [1] -29.40008
```

```
low.loa + qt(zalpha,n-1)*se.loa
```

```
## [1] -14.88536
```

```
plot(x = a, y = d,
ylim= c(-40,100),
xlab = "Average systolic blood pressure (mmHg)",
ylab = "Difference (Machine - Observer)")
abline(h = up.loa)
abline(h = low.loa)
abline(h = bias, lty = 2)
```

Figure 7.4 confirms that the machine tends to over-read systolic blood pressure (positive bias) compared to the observer

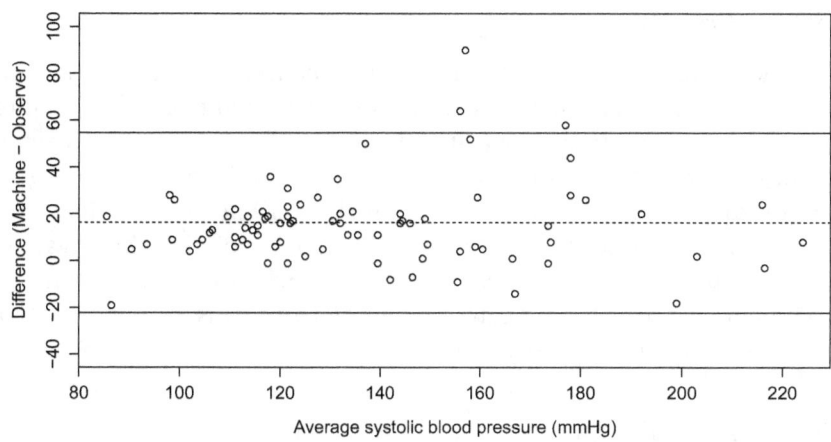

**Fig. 7.4.** Bland–Altman plot of the blood pressure data.

(bias = 16.3 mmHg), and the limits of agreement suggest that 95% of the differences will lie between −22.1 mmHg and +54.7 mmHg. It is fair to say that these limits of agreement render the machine useless for measuring blood pressure in clinical practice, although we note that there is considerable uncertainty regarding the limits of agreement.

## 7.5.2 *Method using logarithmic transformation*

If the variation in the differences depends on the magnitude of the measurement, then we can either take logarithms or compute ratios rather than differences. In this section, we focus on the method using logarithmic transformations.

### 7.5.2.1 *Data requirements*

As before, the data consists of $n$ subjects measured on 2 devices or systems of measurements.

### 7.5.2.2 *Assumptions*

The differences of the log transformed data should satisfy the assumptions in Section 7.5.1.2 – i.e., normality of the differences, uniform bias and standard deviation.

### 7.5.2.3  *Procedure*

First, log transform the new and old measurement data, and then proceed as before. The mean and standard deviation of the difference will now be on the logarithmic scale. The limits of agreement can also be calculated on the log-scale. To get back to the original measurement scale, we need back-transform. The back transformed mean will be the geometric mean of the ratios of the two measurements in the original scale. Similarly, the back-transformed limits of agreement will be the expected range of the ratios of the two measurements on the original scale.

### 7.5.2.4  *Example: Plasma volume*

This example also comes from Bland and Altman (1999). In 99 subjects, plasma volume (expressed as a percentage of normal) was measured using two alternative sets of normal values: the Nadler method and the Hurley method. We now show how to perform the method based on log transformed data using R.

```
data(PlasmaVolume, package = "R4HCR")

# log transformation
ld <- with(PlasmaVolume, log(Nadler) - log(Hurley))
n <- length(ld)
zalpha <- 1 - 0.05/2

# bias (log scale)
(bias <- mean(ld))

## [1] 0.09913773

# limits of agreement (log scale)
(loa <- mean(ld) + c(-1,1)*qnorm(zalpha)*sd(ld))

## [1] 0.05676142 0.14151404

# geometric mean ratio
exp(bias)

## [1] 1.104218
```

```
# limits of agreement (ratio scale)
exp(loa)
```

```
## [1] 1.058403 1.152017
```

The geometric mean of the ratios (Nadler/Hurley) is estimated to be 1.10; that is, the Nadler method, on average, reads 10% higher than the Hurley method. The limits of agreement are between 1.06 and 1.15, which means that the results of the Nadler method exceed those of the Hurley method by 6–15%, 95% of the time. The fact that the lower limit is above 1, indicates that the Nadler consistently returns higher values compared to the Hurley method. More generally, we would anticipate the limits of agreement to include limits below and above 1.

### 7.5.3 Method for non-uniform differences

The log transformation may solve the problem when differences increase with the mean, but it will not work, for example, if the differences decrease with the mean. A more general approach using regression models was proposed by Bland and Altman (1999).

#### 7.5.3.1 Data requirements

The requirements are as per Section 7.5.1.1.

#### 7.5.3.2 Assumptions

The following procedure describes two regression models, one for the differences and one for the residuals from that model. In both cases, we are assuming the relationships between the responses (differences in model 1, and residuals in model 2) and the averages of the differences is linear.

#### 7.5.3.3 Procedure

First calculate the differences ($d$) and averages ($a$) as before. Then proceed to test whether there is a trend in the differences and the variation of the differences over $a$. The trend in differences can be tested using a regression of $d$ on $a$, and the trend in the variation using a regression of the absolute residuals extracted from the first regression model. If no trend is detected in either model, take the bias to be the average value of d ($\bar{d}$) and the standard deviation ($s_d$) for the variation. This is the uniform bias and standard deviation as before (scenario 1). If however, there is a significant trend in the differences but not the residuals, then model the bias as a function of $a$, using the standard deviation of the residuals from model 1 ($\sigma_r$). This is non-uniform bias, uniform standard deviation (scenario 2). If there is also a significant trend detected in the model for the residuals, then also model the variation using an equation. This is non-uniform bias and non-uniform standard deviation (scenario 3). We have therefore, three models for the limits of agreement.

scenario 1: $\bar{d} \pm 1.96 \times s_d$

scenario 2: $(\beta_0 + \beta_1 \times a) \pm 1.96 \times \sigma_r$

scenario 3: $(\beta_0 + \beta_1 \times a) \pm 1.96 \times 1.253 \times (\eta_0 + \eta_1 \times a)$

### 7.5.3.4   *Example: Fat content in milk*

These data are again from Bland and Altman (1999). The data are measurements of the fat content of human milk (g/100 ml) determined through the measurement of glycerol released by enzymatic hydrolysis of triglycerides (Trig) against the standard Gerber method (Gerber).

```
data(Milk, package = "R4HCR")
d <- with(Milk, Trig - Gerber)
a <- with(Milk, (Trig + Gerber)/2)

# regression of difference on the averages

M <- lm(d ~ a)

# The coefficient table
su <- summary(M)
su$coefficients
```

```
##               Estimate Std. Error    t value     Pr(>|t|)
## (Intercept)   0.07904017 0.02906123  2.719781 0.009386433
## a            -0.02827097 0.00944454 -2.993367 0.004559424
```

```
# save the coefficients from the model.
b0 <- coef(M)['(Intercept)']
b1 <- coef(M)['a']
```

```
# SD of the residuals from the first model
sigmar <- sigma(M)
```

```
## [1] 0.08033036
```

The slope coefficient for the bias is estimated to be $-0.02827$ with a $p$-value of 0.0046; this indicates strong evidence of the bias decreasing for higher values of measurement. We now examine whether there is a trend in the residuals.

```
R <- abs(M$residuals)
M2 <- lm(R ~ a)
su <- summary(M2)
```

```
# the slope of the regression line
su$coefficients[2,]
```

```
##    Estimate   Std. Error     t value     Pr(>|t|)
## 0.005166017 0.005863280 0.881079658 0.383173098
```

There is little evidence to suggest a trend in the residuals. So, our equation for the 95% limits of agreement can be written as

$$(0.07904 - 0.02827 \times a) \pm 1.96 \times 0.0803$$

The R code for the Bland-Altman plot with non-uniform limits of agreement are shown below. Figure 7.5 shows how the limits of agreement decrease with the magnitude of measurement.

```
# plotting limits of agreement - no trend in residuals
alpha <- 0.05
uloa <- b0 + b1*a + qnorm(1-alpha/2)*(sigmar)
lloa <- b0 + b1*a - qnorm(1-alpha/2)*(sigmar)
bias <- b0 + b1*a
plot(a,d,
xlab = "Average fat content (g/100 ml)",
ylab = "Difference (Trig - Gerber)")
lines(a,uloa)
lines(a,lloa)
lines(a,bias, lty = 2)
```

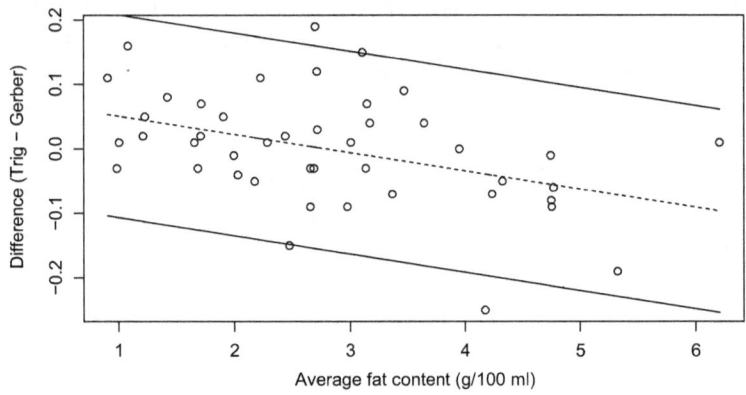

**Fig. 7.5.** Limits of agreement for the two different measurements of milk with non-uniform bias.

### 7.5.4  *Comments*

Sometimes, a limit of agreement study may include multiple measurements on individuals (a repeated-measurement design). It would then be possible to calculate limits of agreement based on either single measurements or the average of multiple measurements. These will invariably lead to different limits of agreement, with the limits based on averages being narrower than those based on individual measurements. When this is the case, the analyst should consult with the clinician to determine what is routinely done in practice: are multiple measurements taken and then averaged, or is it more common to measure only once? For example, it is more common to measure FEV once in clinical practice, and so limits of agreement should reflect this even if the data comes from a repeated measures design. However, there may be examples where the averages of multiple measurements are common, e.g., blood pressure; it might then be preferable to construct limits of agreement based on averages. If the averaging method is deemed appropriate, then the methods described in the previous section can be used, replacing the single new measurement with the average of several new measurements. When single-measurement limits are required but the data contain multiple measurements, then one approach is to select either the first measurement or one at random. There are however methods for utilising all of the data, but these are beyond the scope of this book. The interested reader should look at Section 5 of Bland and Altman (1999) for equations to calculate the limits of agreement in cases where there are equal or unequal number of replicates. An alternative approach for repeated measures uses a variance components model. This model can be fit using the `BA.est()` function from the MethComp package (Carstensen *et al.*, 2008).

## 7.6   Problems and exercises

(1) Use the `PlasmaVolume` data from Section 7.5.2.4 to complete the following tasks:

   (a) Calculate the ratio of the two methods and estimate the mean ratio and limits of agreement.
   (b) Compare your estimates of the bias and limits of agreement to those obtained using the log transform method in Section 7.5.2.
   (c) Finally, create a Bland–Altman plot using the ratio method.

(2) Using the `PEFR` data from Section 7.2.2.4, complete the following tasks:

   (a) Determine which ICC model is most appropriate for these data. Consider the unit of analysis and the different interpretations of agreement and consistency.
   (b) Estimate the agreement ICC and 95% confidence interval. Interpret the value of the ICC.

    (c) Repeat the model to estimate the consistency ICC and con-
fidence interval. Compare with the agreement ICC.

    (d) Finally, investigate whether there is any evidence to sug-
gest these are not true repeat measurements. Explain your
approach and present evidence for or against this hypothesis.

(3) Calculate the reference change value for the PEFR data and
determine what change between two measurements would be
inconsistent with a stable underlying condition.

(4) The following questions focus on comparing the two measurements of cardiac output: thermodilution-derived cardiac output
(TCO) and Fick-derived cardiac output (FCO). Install the package
MethComp and load the CardOutput data. Consult the help page
for more information about the dataset and the variables.

    (a) Plot a scatter plot of TCO vs. FCO and add the line of
equality. What does this plot tell us?

    (b) Carry out a statistical test to compare the means of the TCO
and FCO.

    (c) Produce a histogram and quantile–quantile plot to check
that the difference between two measurements is normally
(approximately) distributed.

    (d) Make a Bland–Altman plot. Add the 95% limits of agree-
ment. Interpret the result.

    (e) Investigate if there is a relationship between the difference
and the mean.

(5) This example comes from Agresti (1996). The following data rep-
resent diagnoses of multiple sclerosis (MS) for two neurologists.
The categories are (1) certain MS, (2) probably MS, (3) possible
MS, and (4) doubtful, unlikely, or definitely not MS.

    (a) Calculate the kappa statistic for these data with linear
weighting. Interpret the result.

    (b) Calculate the kappa statistic using quadratic weights.
Explain the reasoning for doing this.

    (c) Derive the PABAK statistic.

(6) This exercise is based on the hypothetical test–retest data from
Sim and Wright (2005). The data are ratings of movement-
related pain at the shoulder joint.

```
pain <- c("None","Mild","Moderate","Severe")
shoulder <-
matrix(c(15,3,1,1,
4,18,3,2,
4,5,16,4,
1,2,4,17),
ncol=4, byrow=T)
dimnames(shoulder) <- list(pain,pain)
shoulder
```

Use these data to replicate the figures quoted in the paper for the following:

(a) unweighted $\kappa = 0.55$,
(b) linear-weighted $\kappa = 0.61$,
(c) quadratic-weighted $\kappa = 0.67$.

(7) The `blandr.draw()` function from the `blandr` package can be used to draw a Bland–Altman plot. Install the package and reanalyse the data from Section 7.5.1.4.

(8) The `ox` dataset from the `MethComp` package contains data from 61 children who had their blood oxygen content measured at the Children's Hospital in Melbourne, either through a chemical method analysing gases in the blood or by using a pulse oximeter measuring transcutaneously. Use these data to complete the following tasks:

(a) For the blood gas (`CO`) and pulse measurement (`pulse`) separately, check whether there is evidence for the measurement error being proportional to the magnitude of measurement.
(b) Based on the analysis above, calculate either the within-person SD or CV for each measurement.
(c) Calculate a reference change interval for a set-point average of 90. Interpret the result.

(9) The `hba1c` from the `MethComp` package has measurements of HbA1c by three analysers for the determination of HbA1c from venous and capillary blood samples from 38 individuals. Use these data to answer the following questions:

(a) Create a dataset which only consists of the **Tosoh** analyser and the first measurement of the capillary and venous blood sample for each patient.

(b) Calculate the differences and averages of venous and capillary blood HbA1c measurements, and calculate the strength of association.

(c) Derive the 95% limits of agreement for the difference in venous and capillary HbA1c measurements.

# Chapter 8

# Diagnostic accuracy

Diagnostic tests are used in many aspects of patient care and clinical decision-making, helping healthcare professionals decide when to further investigate, initiate treatment, or change a patient's management. It is critical that clinicians are given reliable data about the accuracy of diagnostic tests. To do this, we not only need well-designed diagnostic accuracy studies but also an understanding of how results apply to patients.

**Objectives and learning outcomes**

The objectives for this chapter are to:

- introduce the concept of evaluating the accuracy of diagnostic tests
- outline the most commonly used measures of diagnostic accuracy
- extend methods to tests with ordinal and interval-scaled measurement

After reading this chapter, you should be able to:

- recognise common terms used to describe the accuracy of a test
- use R to evaluate diagnostic tests for binary, ordinal, and interval-scaled data
- carry out Receiver Operating Characteristic (ROC) analysis
- interpret results and assist in clinical decision-making

## 8.1   Introduction

Diagnosis, the process of accurately identifying the cause of disease or ill health is an essential part of clinical practice. In addition to assessing signs and symptoms, doctors may also order blood tests and scans in order to establish a diagnosis. In order to know how useful these tests might be in assisting diagnosis we need to understand how well these tests discriminate between people with a specific disease, and people without a specific disease. In the previous chapter we looked at methods for the case when we want to assess the agreement between two methods, neither of which was assumed to reflect the true condition status of the patient. We now look at methods for comparing tests against the true condition status of the patient.

The accuracy of a test will depend on how well it can separate people with a condition or disease (the *cases*) from those without (non-cases). A perfect test would be able to perfectly separate the cases from non-cases; in other words, the test results of cases would not overlap at all with those of the non-cases. On the other hand, a diagnostic test in which measurements from cases and non-cases completely overlap would be useless. In our experience, most tests fall between these two extremes (see Figure 8.1).

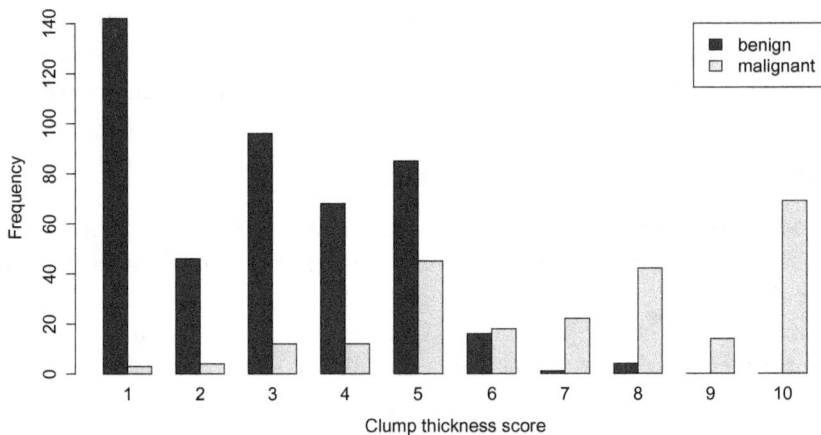

**Fig. 8.1.**   Example of overlap: Although the clump thickness score tends to be higher in malignant tumours and lower in benign tumours, it does not completely discriminate between benign and malignant tumours (data source: `biopsy` dataset (`MASS` package)).

### 8.1.1   *Index test and reference standard*

We use the term *index test* to refer to the test or method under investigation and *reference standard* to refer to the method or test used to define the true condition status. The term test will often refer to a biochemical test such as lateral flow test, but can also used to refer to the predicted probability from an AI algorithm, or the confidence score made by a clinician. Similarly, clinical records, surgery findings, reports, histology or biopsy results, clinical judgement, and combinations of these could determine the reference standard. We assume that the reference standard is the true condition status and does not directly incorporate the index test results. We use the term case to refer to a patient who has the disease of interest according to the reference standard, and a non-case to refer to a patient who does not have that specific disease according to the reference standard.

The index test is usually one of the following three data types, and the approaches to analysis differ accordingly.

- Binary: a pregnancy test or a blood test to detect the presence or absence of antibodies.
- Ordinal: Glasgow Coma Scale or the Breast Imaging Reporting and Data System (BI-RADS).
- Interval-scaled: blood pressure or the level of an antigen in the blood.

### 8.1.2   *Biases*

Diagnostic accuracy studies are prone to several biases that can over- or underestimate the performance of a test. Ideally, the study sample in a diagnostic accuracy study should closely match the clinical setting it is intended for, but often, this is not the case. Table 8.1 provides the names and descriptions of the most common biases encountered in diagnostic accuracy research.

### 8.1.3   *Measures of diagnostic accuracy*

Measures of diagnostic accuracy can be intrinsic or otherwise. Intrinsic measures of accuracy do not depend on the prevalence of cases in the sample being studied. Some measures of diagnostic accuracy such as sensitivity and specificity are intrinsic, while others such as predictive values are not. All of the following measures of diagnostic

**Table 8.1.** Definitions of some common biases found in diagnostic accuracy studies. Adapted from Zhou *et al.* (2002).

| Bias | Description |
| --- | --- |
| Selection bias | The study sample is not representative of the target population |
| Spectrum bias | The study sample does not include the complete spectrum of patient and disease characteristics |
| Imperfect reference standard bias | The reference standard is not 100% accurate |
| Work-up bias | The results of the index test influence the subsequent clinical work-up needed to establish the patient's diagnosis |
| Incorporation bias | The results from the index test are incorporated into the evidence used to establish the reference standard |
| Verification bias | Patients with positive test results are preferentially referred for the reference standard procedure |
| Context bias | When the sample prevalence differs greatly from the population prevalence |

accuracy can be derived from a $2 \times 2$ table of the index test and reference standard as per Table 8.2.

### 8.1.3.1 *Sensitivity and specificity*

Sensitivity is the proportion of cases that are correctly identified by the test:

$$\text{sensitivity} = \frac{a}{a+c}$$

We would expect a test with 80% sensitivity, to detect 80% of people with the condition. The sensitivity is sometimes called the true-positive rate (TPR), although it is not a rate in the usual sense. The complement of sensitivity (1 — sensitivity) is called the false-negative rate (FNR), the proportion of cases not identified or *missed* by the index test.

The specificity of a test is the proportion of non-cases that are correctly identified by the test:

$$\text{specificity} = \frac{d}{b+d}$$

**Table 8.2.** Suggested layout for binary diagnostic data: $a = $ true positives, $b = $ false positives, $c = $ false negatives, $d = $ true negatives, $a + c = $ disease positives (cases), and $b + d = $ disease negatives (non-cases).

|  |  | Reference standard | | Total |
|---|---|---|---|---|
|  |  | Positive | Negative | |
| Index test | Positive | $a$ | $b$ | $a + b$ |
|  | Negative | $c$ | $d$ | $c + d$ |
|  | Total | $a + c$ | $b + d$ | $N$ |

For a test with 90% specificity, we would expect 90% of people without the condition to have negative test result. Specificity is sometimes referred to as the true negative rate (TNR). The complement of specificity (1 − specificity) is called the false positive rate (FPR), the proportion of people who do not have the condition but test positive. A test could have high sensitivity, but it will be of little use in clinical practice if it has low specificity. Ideally, we would like a test to have both a high sensitivity and high specificity.

### 8.1.3.2 *Overall accuracy*

The simplest measure of diagnostic accuracy is the fraction of correct classifications by the index test. As true positives and true negatives are correct classifications, overall accuracy may be defined as the sum of these two divided by the total number of tests:

$$\text{accuracy} = \frac{a + d}{N}$$

Although this measure is intuitive, it is not an intrinsic measure of accuracy, and different index tests with the same accuracy can have very different properties. Suppose a diagnostic test detects 9 out of 10 cases (a sensitivity of 90%) but only correctly identifies 4 out of 10 non-cases (a specificity of 40%). The accuracy of this test is $(4 + 9)/20 = 65\%$. This test has high sensitivity and low false negative rate, and could be used to rule out the condition when the test result is negative (as cases are seldom missed). Contrast this with another test that only detects 4 out of 10 cases and 9 out of 10 non-cases correctly. The accuracy of this second test is also 65%, but it behaves quite differently – you would not be able to rule out disease with this test. The overall accuracy of a test should not be interpreted without the knowledge of the sensitivity and specificity of the test.

### 8.1.3.3 *Positive and negative predictive values*

Predictive values provide a measure of the probability that a patient has or does not have the condition of interest following a positive or negative test result. The positive predictive value (PPV) is the proportion of true positives among all people testing positive:

$$PPV = \frac{a}{a + b}$$

If a test had a PPV of 0.3, we would expect 30% of people who tested positive to have the condition of interest, and 70% not to have the condition. The negative predictive value (NPV) is the proportion of true negatives among all people testing negative:

$$NPV = \frac{d}{c + d}$$

In a test with an NPV of 0.9, we would expect 90% of people who tested negative not to have the condition, and 10% to have the condition. The predictive values, unlike sensitivity and specificity, depend on the sample prevalence, which may not reflect the prevalence in the population. This can be explained as follows. The predictive values are the proportions of row totals and so they are affected by sample prevalance. In contrast, sensitivity and specificity are proportions of column total and so they will not be affected by the sample prevalence.

### 8.1.3.4 *Diagnostic likelihood ratios*

The diagnostic likelihood is the ratio of probabilities of the same test result occurring in the cases compared to the non-cases. As we have seen, the probability of a positive test among cases is called the sensitivity or the TPR. The probability of a positive test amongst non-cases is the FPR. The positive likelihood ratio is therefore:

$$\text{positive likelihood ratio } (LR^+) = TPR/FPR$$

The negative likelihood ratio is the probability of a negative test among cases (FNR) compared to the probability of a negative test result among non-cases (TNR). The negative likelihood ratio is therefore:

$$\text{negative likelihood ratio (LR}^-) = \text{FNR/TNR}$$

A test with 90% sensitivity and 40% specificity would have $\text{LR}^+ = 0.9/(1-0.4) = 1.25$ and $\text{LR}^- = (1-0.9)/0.4 = 0.25$. This means that someone with the disease is 1.25 times as likely to test positive than someone without the disease and 0.25 times as likely to test negative than someone without the disease. If $\text{LR}^+$ or $\text{LR}^-$ is close to 1, then it means that people with or without a disease are equally likely to test positive or negative respectively and the test cannot discriminate between cases and non-cases. The next section will discuss how the prevalence of disease in the population can be modified, based on the likelihood ratios of the test.

### 8.1.3.5 *Pre-test to post-test probability*

We now show how we can use likelihood ratios to calculate the probability of disease after a test result (post-test probability). The calculation requires a pre-test odds of disease and a likelihood ratio. If these are taken directly from a sample the post-test probability will be the same as the predictive values (PPV and NPV). However, this method can be generalised to other prevalence estimates and likelihood ratios. The post-test odds are found by multiplying the pre-test odds by the likelihood ratio.

$$\text{pre-test odds} \times \text{LR} = \text{post-test odds}$$

if the test is both sensitive and specific ($\text{LR}^+ > 10$ and $\text{LR}^- < 0.1$), the post-test probability will increase substantially following a positive test result and become reduced significantly if the test result is negative. A poorly performing test will likely only slightly change the pre-test probability.

For example, suppose the prevalence of a condition in a specific population is known to be 1%. We will use this as a pre-test probability. The pre-test odds for any person from that population are, therefore, 1/99. Further, assume that the diagnostic test being used has sensitivity and specificity of 90%. Now, if the test comes back positive, we multiply the pre-test odds by the positive likelihood ratio, and if the test is negative, we multiply the pre-test odds by the negative likelihood ratio. The positive likelihood ratio is 9. The post-test odds are, therefore, $1/99 \times 9 = 1/11$. The odds of the disease being present are nine times greater following a positive test. For a negative test result and a negative likelihood ratio of $1/9$, our post-test odds are $1/99 \times 1/9 = 1/891$. The odds of the condition being present have significantly reduced following a negative test. To aid interpretation further, we often convert the odds back to probabilities. The following R code shows how this can be done:

```
# sensitivity, specificity
sn <- 0.9
sp <- 0.9

# likelihood ratios
pos.likelihood.ratio <- sn/(1-sp)
neg.likelihood.ratio <- (1-sn)/sp

pre.test.prob <- 0.01
pre.test.odds <- (pre.test.prob/(1 -pre.test.prob))

# if the test result is positive
pos.post.odds <- pre.test.odds * pos.likelihood.ratio

# if the test result is negative
neg.post.odds <- pre.test.odds * neg.likelihood.ratio

# post-test probability of disease after a positive test
pos.post.odds/(1 + pos.post.odds)

## [1] 0.08333333

# post-test probability of disease after a negative test
neg.post.odds/(1 + neg.post.odds)

## [1] 0.001121076
```

In our example, the pre-test probability was 1% before the test was carried out and a positive test would increase this probability of disease to 8.3%. A negative test result would move the pre-test probability from 1% to 0.1%. Even though this test has high sensitivity and high specificity, it is by no means certain that this person has the disease after a positive test. Similarly, a negative test does not completely rule out the probability of disease, but it certainly makes it less likely. These results, and other similar examples, are very surprising to most people when they encounter them; there is a tendency to think that the post-test probability would be high if a test has high sensitivity. The post test probability depends strongly on the pre-test probability, much like the predictive values depend strongly on the sample prevalence. The sensitivity, specificity and likelihood ratios are not affected in the same way (see later exercise).

### 8.1.3.6 *Diagnostic odds ratio*

Another measure that combines sensitivity and specificity, and does not depend on the prevalence is diagnostic odds ratio (DOR). It is the ratio of the odds of testing positive among people with the condition to the odds of testing positive among people without the disease. It is equivalent to the ratio of likelihood ratios (Glas *et al.*, 2003):

$$\text{DOR} = \frac{\text{TPR/FNR}}{\text{FPR/TNR}} \equiv \frac{\text{LR}^+}{\text{LR}-} = \frac{ad}{bc}$$

A DOR of 1 would indicate the test is no better than chance at discriminating people with and without the condition. DOR > 1 indicates the test has some diagnostics value. Higher DORs are better. Our example has DOR = 81. DOR <1 means the tests is in the wrong direction.

### 8.1.3.7 *Youden's index*

Youden's index is another measure that reflects the likelihood of a positive result among patients with versus without the condition. It can be written as follows:

$$\text{Youden's index} = \text{sensitivity} + \text{specificity} - 1$$

A diagnostic test that is no better than chance will have a Youden's index of 0. In contrast, if the test has near-perfect sensitivity and specificity, Youden's will be close to 1. Note that while Youden's and the DOR are intrinsic measures, they can have similar or equal values for tests with very different properties. A test with sensitivity 90% and specificity 40% has the same DOR of 6 and Youden' index of 0.3 as a test with sensitivity 40% and specificity 90%.

## 8.2    Methods for binary data

A diagnostic test will often produce either a negative or positive result. A rapid pregnancy and lateral flow test are such examples. As we also assume that the reference standard result takes one of two mutually exclusive states (e.g., either positive or negative), there are four combinations of index test and reference standard (see Table 8.2).

### 8.2.1    *Data requirements*

In the *complete* study design, each subject receives the index and reference standard test. In other designs, only a subset of patients receive the reference standard. These are susceptible to verification bias (see Table 8.1). When only the test positives undergo the reference standard evaluation, we can only be sure of who is true positive and false positive, and only estimate the PPV.

### 8.2.2    *Assumptions*

The reference standard is assumed to be true condition status of the patients. An arguably more critical assumption is that the reference standard result and index test were derived independently. Incorporation and work-up bias, if present, are likely to lead to overstating the accuracy of a diagnostic test.

### 8.2.3    *Procedures*

Most diagnostic accuracy measures are based on probabilities or proportions. We can therefore use functions or tests suitable for proportions to estimate confidence intervals for the measures that are proportions (such as sensitivity, specificity, PPV, and NPV).

Examples include `binom.test()`, which uses the exact method for confidence intervals, and `prop.test()`, which employs the Clopper–Pearson method.

```
# For sensitivity & exact CIs
binom.test(x = a, n = a + c)

# For specificity & Clopper-Pearson CIs
prop.test(x = d, n  = b+d)

# PPV Clopper-Pearson CIs
binom.test(x = a, n  = a+c)

# NPV & Clopper-Pearson CIs
prop.test(x = d, n  = c+d)
```

Accuracy measures that are ratios (e.g., likelihood ratios) require a different method for calculating confidence intervals (see the following section). In the case of a complete design, we can obtain a full set of metrics and corresponding confidence intervals using the `epi.tests()` function from the `epiR` library. This calculates 18 different statistical measures of diagnostic accuracy from a $2 \times 2$ table. The default method for confidence intervals is the 'exact' method, in which the calculation of sensitivity and specificity is the same as using `binom.test()` function.

```
# tb is a table with tp's in top right cell

da.stats <- epiR::epi.tests(tb)

# All 18 stats
da.stats$detail
```

### 8.2.4  *Example 1*

The Pathfinder study was a prospective cohort study of a multi-cancer early detection test (MCED) (Schrag *et al.*, 2023). Among 6661 adults who were screened, 92 were detected with a cancer signal

**Table 8.3.** Results of the Pathfinder study (Schrag *et al.*, 2023).

| | | Diagnostic evaluation | | |
| | | Positive | Negative | Total |
|---|---|---|---|---|
| MCED test | Positive | 35 | 57 | 92 |
| | Negative | – | – | – |
| | Total | – | – | – |

(index test positive) and referred for further investigation. Of the 92 people, 35 were true positives and 57 were false positives. As only the test positives were followed up with diagnostic evaluation (the reference standard), only the positive predictive value can be estimated (see Table 8.3).

We can calculate the exact confidence intervals for the Pathfinder study as follows:

```
# Exact method
# PATHFINDER
# PPV = tp/(tp + fp)

bt <- binom.test(x = 35, n = 35 + 57)

# Estimated PPV  = 35/92
bt$estimate

## probability of success
##               0.3804348

# 95% confidence interval
bt$conf.int

## [1] 0.2811766 0.4876165
## attr(,"conf.level")
## [1] 0.95
```

The positive predictive value of the test is estimated to be 38% with 95% confidence interval of 28–49%.

## 8.2.5  *Example 2*

These data are from a screening trial conducted in Dschang (West Cameroon) between February 2019 and March 2020. Women aged 30–49 were invited to participate in a free cervical cancer screening campaign. Primary HPV-based screening was followed by a pelvic exam for visual assessment (viewing the cervix with the naked eye to identify colour changes on the cervix) and then cervical biopsy and endocervical curettage. The study aimed to assess whether the use, in addition to regular visual inspection, of images captured using a smartphone could improve the detection of precancerous lesions or cancer. For this example, we focus on the digitally enhanced visual inspection (D-VIA/VILI) version of the index test. The reference standard was classified negative if the cervix was without cervical intraepithelial neoplasia (CIN) or was low-grade (CIN1) and positive if the cervix had high grade CIN (CIN2 or CIN3, adenocarcinoma in-situ (AIS) or cancer). The Smartphone dataset contains the outcomes of 188 HPV-positive women who consented to take part in the study.

```
data(Smartphone, package = "R4HCR")

# this is the index test of interest
indx <- Smartphone$smart_via
levels(indx)

## [1] "negative" "positive"

# and the reference test.
refst <- Smartphone$CIN2plus
levels(refst)

## [1] "<CIN2" "CIN2+"
```

The CIN2plus variable takes one of two levels; <CIN2 (reference standard negative) and CIN2+ (reference standard positive). The smart_via variable represents the index test result and is either negative or positive. Before proceeding with the analysis, we first use the relevel() function to ensure our 2 × 2 table has index test and reference standard positive in the top left corner of the table.

```
# indx test
indx <- relevel(indx, ref = "positive")

# reference test
refst <- relevel(refst, ref = "CIN2+")

# create a 2-way table
tb <- table(index = indx, reference_std = refst)
tb

##                reference_std
## index          CIN2+ <CIN2
##    positive      23   106
##    negative       2    49

da.stats <- epiR::epi.tests(tb)
dts <- da.stats$detail

# rows 3,4 ,11 and 12 give sensitivity, specificity
# positive and negative likelihood ratios
dts[c(3,4,11,12),]

##     statistic        est        lower       upper
## 3          se 0.9200000 0.73969416 0.9901604
## 4          sp 0.3161290 0.24388067 0.3955667
## 11    lr.pos 1.3452830 1.14920061 1.5748220
## 12    lr.neg 0.2530612 0.06564779 0.9755085
```

The sensitivity of the enhanced digital visual inspection is $23/25 = 92.0\%$ with a 95% confidence interval of 74.0–99.0%. The uncertainty around this estimate is due to the relatively low number of cases ($n = 25$). The test is, however, not very specific for CIN2+; the specificity is $106/154 = 31.6\%$. The 95% confidence for the specificity is more precise than the sensitivity because there are more non-cases ($n = 154$) than cases. This is often the case in diagnostic studies. The positive likelihood ratio estimate of 1.35 suggests that a positive test is 35% more likely in a woman with CIN2+ than in a woman who doesn't have CIN2+. The negative likelihood ratio tells us that a negative test is $1 - 0.2530612 = 74.7\%$ less likely in a woman with CIN2+ than in a woman without CIN2+.

## 8.3 Comparing two diagnostic tests

The sensitivity or specificity of two tests can be compared in independent or paired samples. For independent samples, one group of patients receive one index test and the reference standard, and another group of patients receive the second index test and the reference standard. In the paired design, each patient undergoes both index tests and the reference standard. For the independent study design, we can use a function such as `prop.test()` to compare sensitivity or specificity, but for dependent or paired samples we need to account for the dependency. We now show how to analyse sensitivity and specificity in paired samples.

### 8.3.1 *Data requirements*

In the paired design, each patient has a result for index test 1, a result for index test 2, and a reference standard classification.

### 8.3.2 *Assumptions*

The two groups (index test 1 and index test 2) are from the same individuals.

### 8.3.3 *Procedures*

To compare sensitivity, we would cross-tabulate the two index test results in subjects who were reference standard positive. To compare specificity, we construct a two-way table of the two index test results in subjects who were reference standard negative.

```
# to compare sensitivities we take only cases
# E.g.
cases <- subset(data, RefStd == "Positives")

# index tests being compared
indx1 <- cases$indextest1
indx2 <- cases$indextest2
```

```
# 2-way table
tb2 <- table(indx1, indx2)

# McNemar test using correct = F
mcnemar.test(tb2)
```

The standard `mcnemar.test()` function only calculates a $p$-value for the comparison and does not supply a confidence interval for the difference. However, `mcnemar.exact()` calculates a confidence interval but does so for the conditional odds ratio rather than the differences in proportions. If the number of discordant results $(b + c)$ is less than 20, then an exact test may be better (Zhou *et al.*, 2002), irrespective of the need for a confidence interval.

### 8.3.4    *Example*

In the smartphone study, they wanted to compare the accuracy of a combined approach (naked-eye and digital VIA) with a traditional naked-eye approach. The study is paired, as the two index tests are evaluated on the same set of patients. We replicate their analysis by comparing the sensitivity of both methods to detect CIN2+.

```
cases <- subset(Smartphone, CIN2plus == "CIN2+")

# index tests being compared
indx1 <- cases$smart_via
indx1 <- relevel(indx1, ref = "positive")

indx2 <- cases$naked_via
indx2 <- relevel(indx2, ref = "positive")

# 2-way table
(tb2 <- table(indx1, indx2))

##              indx2
## indx1      positive negative
##    positive        20        3
##    negative         0        2
```

```
# using correct = F
# to match the analysis in the paper
mcnemar.test(tb2, correct = F)

##
## McNemar's Chi-squared test
##
## data:  tb2
## McNemar's chi-squared = 3, df = 1, p-value = 0.08326

# exact test (not run)
#install.packages("exact2x2")
#library(exact2x2)
#mcnemar.exact(tb2)
```

For the 25 reference standard positive cases, 20 were positive for both methods, and two were negative for both. For three patients the naked visual assessment was negative, whilst the smartphone method was correctly positive. Although the sensitivity of the smartphone method in the study is superior to the naked visual assessment, a *p*-value of 0.083 does not provide overwhelming evidence for a true difference in the sensitivities of the two tests. The McNemar test statistic depends on the number of discordant results. It is calculated as $(c - b)/2$, which will tend to zero when there is an equal number of discordant results and will be large (and significant) if one test performs better or worse. A test comparing specificities can be done by selecting only the women without high grade CIN or cancer.

## 8.4   Methods for ordinal-scale data

Some diagnostic tests produce ordinal-scale results. These often involve subjective judgement such as the reading of images by a radiologist. A typical ordinal rating scale would look like the following:

(1) definitely not present,
(2) probably not present,
(3) possibly present,
(4) probably present,
(5) definitely present.

As before, we assume that the reference standard is binary. The general approach to dealing with ordinal data is to evaluate the diagnostic accuracy at each possible threshold. By doing this, it is then possible to determine a best threshold for use in clinical practice.

### 8.4.1   Data requirements

The function we recommend for ordinal data, allows the user to enter data in two ways. (1) A vector of index test results in the cases, and another vector of index test results in the non-cases, and (2) a vector that identifies which patients are cases and which are non-cases (responses), and a vector containing the index test results (predictor).

### 8.4.2   Assumptions

The index test measurements or interpretations can be meaningfully ranked in magnitude, and the decision thresholds are the same for cases and non-cases. The first assumption should follow if the data are genuinely ordinal rather than nominal. The latter assumption applies mainly to the case of subjective judgements (as opposed to biochemical test results).

### 8.4.3   Procedures

The analysis of ordinal-scale index test data proceeds by creating multiple $2 \times 2$ tables, each one corresponding to a different threshold. At each threshold, measures of accuracy are calculated. For example, the BI-RAD index test in Table 8.4 can be split into four $2 \times 2$ tables corresponding to four thresholds. The first threshold would reclassify the lowest grade (normal) as negative, and all higher grades (2–5) as positive. When the index test is classified in this way, the sensitivity is 29/30 as 29 of the cases is test positive, and the specificity is 9/30 as 9 non-cases are test negative. If we now move the threshold up, so that negative is categories 1–2, and positives are categories 3–5, the sensitivity is still 29/30 but the specificity is 11/30. We can move the threshold up two more times, calculating sensitivity and specificity at each point. By convention, two additional thresholds are also included, corresponding to 'always negative' and 'always

**Table 8.4.** Results of workstation-displayed digitised-film mammogram (BI-RAD-System Reader response) (Zhou *et al.*, 2002).

|  | Cancer status | |
|---|---|---|
|  | Present | Absent |
| Normal (1) | 1 | 9 |
| Benign (2) | 0 | 2 |
| Prob. Benign (3) | 6 | 11 |
| Suspicious (4) | 11 | 8 |
| Malignant (5) | 12 | 0 |
| Total | 30 | 30 |

positive'. The `roc()` function from the pROC package can be used to perform these calculations.

The `roc()` function requires individual-level data, so if the data are in table form, they will need to be de-aggregated. This is easily achieved using the `rep()` function. For example, for the mammography data, we could do the following:

```
# For the cases and controls format
# present = cases, absent = controls
cases <- rep(1:5, times = c(1,0,6,11,12))
controls <- rep(1:5, times = c(9,2,11,8,0))
```

When using the `roc()` function, it is good practice to specify the 'direction' of the index test result. This refers to whether lower or higher values of the index test result are associated with increasing likelihood of disease. For example, we associate higher BI-RADS grades with a higher likelihood of cancer being present. In our experience, it is common for higher values of the index test to be associated with an increased likelihood of disease, but this isn't always the case. The `roc()` function takes a guess if you don't specify the direction by comparing the test results in cases and controls, and whilst this is often correct, we think it should be set explicitly. The direction argument takes one of two arguments;

direction = "<" when the test results in the non-cases are expected to be lower than the test results in the cases.

`direction = ">"` when the test results in the non-cases are expected to be higher than the test results in the cases.

If higher scores are more likely to come from cases than non-cases, we would expect the median of the test values in the cases to be higher than the median in the non-cases. In the mammography example, the median reader response was 8 in the cancer cases and 6 in the non-cases. As we expect the scores to be lower in the non-cases, we specify `direction = "<"` in the syntax.

```r
pROC::roc(controls = controls,
cases = cases,
direction = "<")

# For the predictor and response format
response <- c(rep(0, length(controls)),
rep(1,length(cases)))
predictor <- c(controls, cases)

pROC::roc(response ~ predictor,
direction = "<")

# or
pROC::roc(response = response,
predictor = predictor,
direction = "<")
```

### 8.4.4  Example

We illustrate the ordinal data method using data from a reader study on pneumothoraces (PTX's). In this study, readers were asked to give their confidence rating in the presence of a pneumothorax (PTX) on X-ray. The PTXII data contains one of the reader's confidence scores (predictor) and a reference standard outcome representing the presence or absence of pneumothorax (response).

```r
data(PTXII, package = "R4HCR")
roc1 <- pROC::roc(response ~ predictor,
data = PTXII,
direction = "<",
percent = T)
```

```
## Setting levels: control = 0, case = 1
data.frame(thresholds = roc1$thresholds,
sns = roc1$sensitivities,
spec = roc1$specificities,
Youden = roc1$sensitivities - (100-roc1$specificities))
```

```
##    thresholds        sns        spec      Youden
## 1        -Inf  100.00000    0.00000    0.00000
## 2         1.5   96.55172   30.96774   27.51947
## 3         2.5   88.27586   76.12903   64.40489
## 4         3.5   73.10345   96.12903   69.23248
## 5         4.5   71.03448   96.12903   67.16352
## 6         5.5   68.27586   98.06452   66.34038
## 7         6.5   60.00000   98.06452   58.06452
## 8         7.5   46.20690   98.70968   44.91657
## 9         Inf    0.00000  100.00000    0.00000
```

The threshold with the largest Youden's index can be used to define a diagnostic threshold. The output shows that Youden's index is maximised when the score is 3.5 (Youden's index = 69.2). We could therefore define 3.5 as a threshold and dichotmise the scores accordingly. All scores greater than 3.5 are called positive, and all scores less than or equal to 3.5 are called negative. At this threshold we would expect this test to have sensitivity of 73% and specificity of 96%.

## 8.5 Methods for interval-scaled data

When the index test result is interval-scaled, we can generalise the approach used for ordinal data and consider the test's accuracy at multiple thresholds. This is often referred to as a receiver operating characteristic (ROC) analysis, which focuses on a graphic called the ROC curve.

### 8.5.1 *Receiver operating characteristic curve*

The ROC curve is a graphic representation of the diagnostic accuracy of ordinal or interval-scaled diagnostic tests. The $x$ and $y$ coordinates are 1 − specificity and sensitivity, and points represent the sensitivity and 1 − specificity of the test at different thresholds. The individual points are often joined using a step function to form an ROC curve.

Most ROC curves in the literature are empirical ROC curves (step-like in appearance), smooth ROC curves exist but are seldom used. Some ROC curves have a 'hook' − these are called 'improper' ROC curves. Improper ROC curves can indicate that there is more variability in the test result in patients without the condition than with the condition. An improper ROC curve warrants checking the data for errors and outlying values.

### 8.5.2   *Interpreting the ROC curve*

Figure 8.2 shows how to interpret individual points in ROC space. Thresholds corresponding to high sensitivity and high specificity lie in the top-left hand corner of the plot, whereas points close to the line

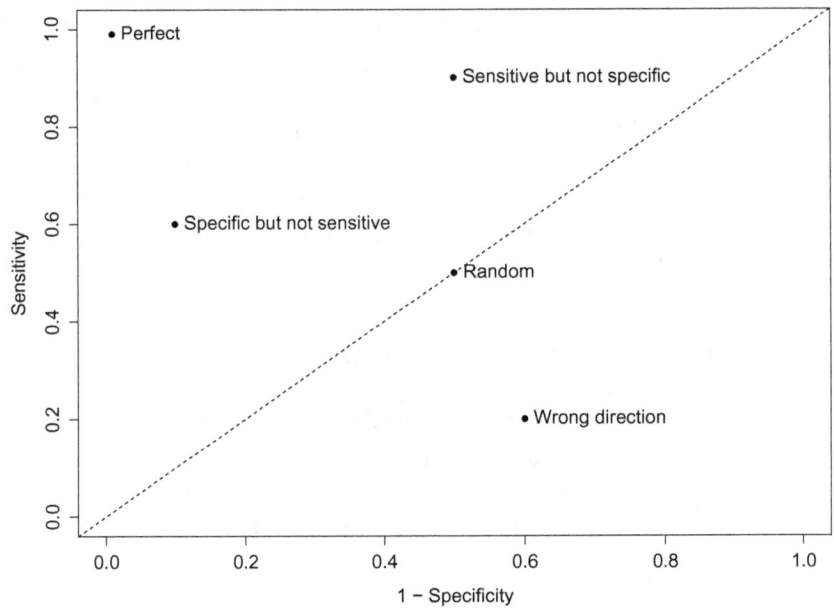

**Fig. 8.2.**   Thresholds that are no better than chance fall along the diagonal line. Thresholds associated with 100% sensitivity and specificity sit in the north-west corner, thresholds that are specific but not sensitive reside in the southwest, whereas sensitive but not specific inhabit the northeast corner of the plot. Points below the line may correspond to errors in case definition, wrong index test direction, or abnormally poor performance.

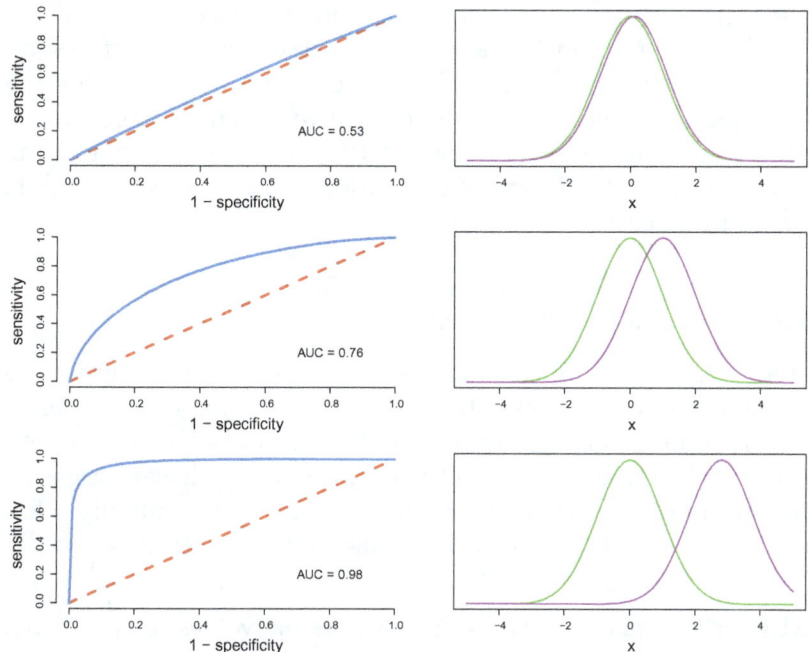

**Fig. 8.3.** Receiver operating characteristic (ROC). Area under the ROC curve (AUC) statistic and density curves representing the index test result distributions in cases and non-cases. The index test results are assumed to come from two normal distributions with equal variance 1, but with the mean shifted in the cases by 0.1 sd (top panels), 1 sd (middle panels), and 2.8 sd (bottom panels). The ROC curve, and AUC reflect the increasing shift in means (separation) between cases and non-case index test distributions.

of equality represent tests no better than chance. Points below the line should be checked to see whether an error in case/non-case definition has been made or whether the direction has been mispecified. When the distribution of test results in the cases overlaps entirely with the distribution of test results in controls, the ROC curve will fall entirely along the chance diagonal and have an area under the curve (AUC) of 0.5 (Figure 8.3, top panels). Such a test will be no better than a coin flip and unusable in clinical practice. When the distribution of cases and controls is separated somewhat (but still overlaps), the ROC curve curves away from the chance diagonal and towards the northwest corner. This curve will have $0.5 < \text{AUC} < 1$ (Figure 8.3, middle panels). Such tests will have some ability to discriminate between cases and non-cases and may be useful clinically in the right setting. As the ROC curve moves closer to the left-hand corner, the AUC tends to 1, and the distribution of test results of cases and controls is separated, with minimal overlap (Figure 8.3, bottom panels). These tests will perform very well as diagnostic tools in clinical settings. In summary, the ROC curve and the area under the curve reflect the degree of separation between the test results of cases and non-cases.

### 8.5.3   *Area under the curve*

The area under the ROC curve is, foremost, a global measure of a test's ability to discriminate between cases and non-cases. There are, however, other interpretations. The AUC can also be interpreted as the probability that a test result from a randomly chosen case is more indicative of disease than the result from another randomly selected non-case. The AUC also has the following interpretations:

- AUC = Average sensitivity for all possible values of specificity.
- AUC = Average specificity for all possible values of sensitivity.

Because sensitivity and specificity are independent of the sample prevalence, so is the ROC curve – and by implication, so is the AUC. The ROC curve is also scale-invariant to monotonic transformations of the test results. If we add or multiply the score any number (other than zero), the ROC curve will not change. This is because the empirical curve depends only on the ranks of observation, not the actual magnitude of the test results. The ROC method is particularly useful for comparing two or more tests. Disadvantages include the fact that the AUC has no direct clinical interpretation and can consist of regions that are not clinically relevant. In addition, it is possible for index tests to have the same AUC value but perform differently at different points of the curve.

### 8.5.4   *Empirical ROC curve*

An empirical ROC curve estimates the sensitivity and specificity pairs at all possible thresholds and uses a step function to draw an ROC curve.

### 8.5.4.1  *Data requirements*

As for ordinal data.

### 8.5.4.2  *Assumptions*

The assumptions of the ROC analysis for interval data are the same as those for ordinal data.

### 8.5.4.3  *Procedures*

We use the `roc()` function from the `pROC` package for ROC analysis of interval-scaled data. The AUC and a 95% confidence interval are also available from this function. A smooth ROC curve can be fitted using a binormal model (not to be confused with a binomial).

### 8.5.4.4  *Example*

Kim *et al.* (2022) set out to evaluate the effect of the AI tool on the performance of radiologists and pulmonologists in risk stratification of indeterminate pulmonary nodules (IPNs) on chest CT scans. The AI tool gave a score representing the likelihood of cancer (from 0 to 100). The `IPNs` dataset consists of the score and classification outcomes for 200 CT scans. The R-code below performs the ROC analysis and plot the ROC curve (Figure 8.4). As a higher score is associated with a higher risk of cancer, we specify `direction = "<"`.

```
data(IPNs, package = "R4HCR")

# The ROC analysis
rc1 <- pROC::roc(cancer ~ rating,
data = IPNs,
direction = "<")

## Setting levels: control = 0, case = 1

# Area under the curve.
pROC::auc(rc1)

## Area under the curve: 0.7791

# 95% CI for AUC
pROC::ci.auc(rc1)

## 95% CI: 0.7119-0.8463 (DeLong)
plot(rc1, legacy.axes = TRUE, grid = TRUE)
```

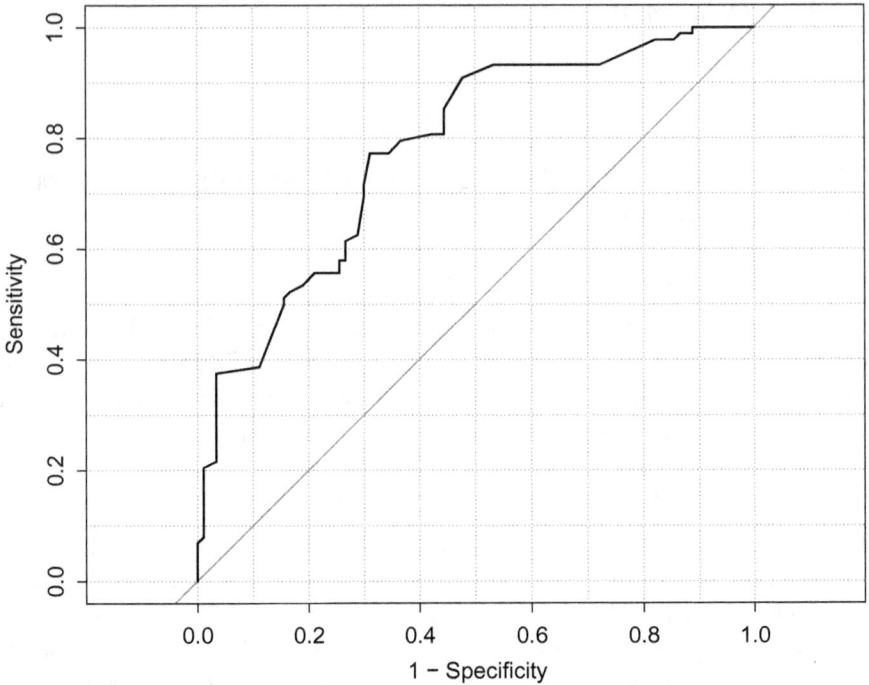

**Fig. 8.4.** An empirical receiver operating characteristic (ROC) curve of the nodule data. The legacy axes option is selected ($x$ axis is 1 – specificity) and a chance diagonal is superimposed to aid interpretation.

The AUC (95% CI) for the AI algorithm (without a radiologist) is 77.9% (71.2–84.6%). This is interpreted as follows: if we randomly choose a case and a non-case, the AI tool is likely to identify the case 77.9% of the time. The confidence interval confirms that there is strong evidence that the performance of the AI algorithm is better than chance as it excludes the an AUC of 50%.

### 8.5.5   *Smooth ROC curve*

There are several methods for smoothing ROC curves. The `roc()` function default is the **binormal** method, which works by fitting a linear model to the quantiles of the sensitivities and specificities.

This is perhaps the simplest approach and seems to work well in most situations. Other methods use the kernal density estimation.

### 8.5.5.1  *Procedures*

Here we provide code to do the default binormal smoothing. The full extent of options for smoothing can be found on the help page `?pROC::smooth`.

### 8.5.5.2  *Example*

We now fit a smooth ROC curve to the nodule data and re-estimate the AUC.

```
# Smooth ROC curve
rc2 <- pROC::roc(cancer ~ rating,
data = IPNs,
smooth = TRUE,
direction = "<")

## Setting levels: control = 0, case = 1

# Area under the curve.
pROC::auc(rc2)

## Area under the curve: 0.7785

# 95% CI for AUC
pROC::ci.auc(rc2)

## 95% CI: 0.7104-0.841 (2000 stratified bootstrap
   replicates)
```

The effect of smoothing is clearly visible from the ROC plot (Figure 8.5). For these data, the AUC and 95% confidence interval are largely unchanged from the equivalent estimates from the empirical (unsmoothed) ROC.

To calculate the sensitivity at a particular false positive rate for the smoothed ROC curve, we can do:

```
a <- rc2$model$coefficients[1]
b <- rc2$model$coefficients[2]
```

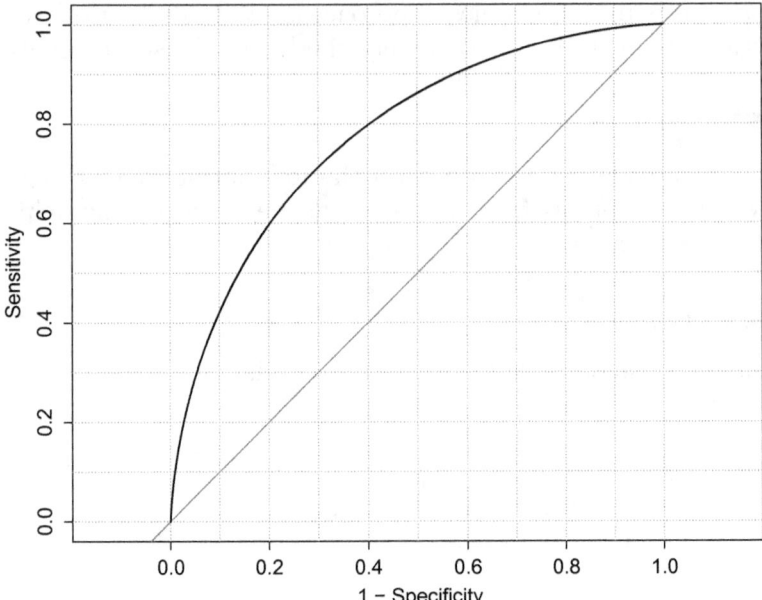

**Fig. 8.5.** Smoothed ROC curve of the nodule data, with legacy axes and chance diagonal superimposed.

```
# 'Sensitivity for false positive rate 0.2 can be
    calculated from:
pnorm(a + b * qnorm(1-0.2))

##   (Intercept)
##   0.5963668
```

## 8.6   Comparing ROC curves

As we might want to compare the sensitivity or specificity of two diagnostic tests, we might also want to compare two ROC curves using a hypothesis testing approach. We can do this in a number of ways:

- Test the partial or whole ROC area.
- Test sensitivity/specificity at fixed specificity/sensitivity.
- Test if the ROC curves are identical for all possible thresholds.

### 8.6.1   *Data requirements*

For a paired design, data consist of response (the reference standard) and two predictors (one for each index test). Alternatively, for independent designs, the data are two sets of corresponding response-predictor variables.

### 8.6.2   *Assumptions*

Knowing whether the comparison is between two correlated (or paired) or uncorrelated (unpaired) designs is important. If not specified in the `roc()` function will try to detect paired status if it exists.

#### 8.6.2.1   *Procedure 1*

There are three methods available in the `roc.test()` function at the time of writing. The first, `method="DeLong"`, is the default method for all comparisons except partial AUC smoothed curves and curves with a different direction. It should not be used when the ROC curves have different directions (as per our example), and an error will be printed. Partial areas will be ignored in Delong's method. This method produces a confidence interval for the difference in AUC's and is therefore preferred over the other methods when applied. The `method = "bootstrap"` approach is the most flexible and can be used for smooth curves with different directions and partial areas.

```
# Assuming r1 and r2 are two fitted ROC curves as before.

# compare entire ROC area.
pROC::roc.test(r1,r2)

# comparison of areas restricted to
   0.7 < specificity <= 1
pROC::roc.test(r1, r2,
reuse.auc=FALSE,
partial.auc=c(1, 0.7),
partial.auc.focus="sp")
```

## 8.6.2.2 *Procedure 2*

Test sensitivities at fixed specificity can be tested as can specificities at fixed sensitivity. The R code is as follows:

```
# compare sensitivity @ specificity  = 0.9
pROC::roc.test(r1, r2,
method="specificity", specificity = 0.9)

# compare specificity @ sensitivity  = 0.85
pROC::roc.test(r1, r2,
method="sensitivity", sensitivity = 0.85)
```

## 8.6.2.3 *Procedure 3*

This approach tests the hypothesis that the two curves are identical for all operating points, unlike the previous methods, which test the equality of full or partial areas under the ROC curves. The method proposed by Venkatraman and Begg (1996) is based on a permutation test and has a counterpart for paired diagnostic data and unpaired diagnostic data. Due to the nature of the test, we have an additional assumption: the index tests possess equivalent diagnostic information under the null hypothesis.

```
# increase boot.n for more precision
rt <- pROC::roc.test(r1,r2,
method = "venkatraman", boot.n=1000)
rt$p.value
```

## 8.6.2.4 *Example*

We illustrate Procedure 2 (sensitivity for fixed specificity) using the OXFIT dataset of two biochemical tests: albumin excretion and C-reactive protein (CRP). We note that albumin tends to be higher in the non-cases than in those with cancer, and so we specify `direction = ">"`. CRP is lower in the non-cases than in the cancers, and so we specify the direction as `direction = "<"`.

```
set.seed(1)

r1 <- pROC::roc(cancer ~ albumin,
data = OXFIT, direction=">")
r2 <- pROC::roc(cancer ~ crp,
data = OXFIT, direction="<")

tst <- pROC::roc.test(r1, r2,
method="specificity", specificity = 0.9)
```

The $p$-value (0.15) for this specificity test of albumin and CRP suggests there is little evidence for a difference in the true sensitivities. Although, a point estimate for the difference is not given, the sign of the $D$ test statistic does indicate which sensitivity is higher. In this example $D$ is negative as the sensitivity of albumin is lower than the sensitivity of CRP. It can be useful to plot the two curves, and draw a vertical line at the level of specificity used in the test to illustrate the difference.

## 8.7 Finding optimal thresholds

Diagnostic tests that produce interval or ordinal scaled results will often need to be dichotomised at a particular threshold. As a test's performance will vary at different thresholds, one threshold may be better than any other in some objective sense. We now look at how to do this in R.

### 8.7.1 *Data requirements*

An empirical or smoothed ROC curve. Note that not all functions and options can be used with smoothed curves.

### 8.7.2 *Procedures*

There are several criteria, but two commonly used methods for establishing optimal thresholds are the point on the ROC curve closest to the top-left corner (0,1) and Youden's index

(Perkins and Schisterman, 2006). The 'closest to the top-left corner' of the ROC is equivalent to minimising

$$(1 - \text{sensitivity})^2 + r \times (1 - \text{specificity})^2$$

For Youden's index, we would look to maximise

$$\text{sensitivity} + r \times \text{specificity} - 1$$

where the weight $r$ is $(1 - p)/(c \times p)$, $p$ is the prevalence of disease or condition, and $c$ is the cost representing the relative loss costs of a false negative classification compared to a false positive. If $p = 0.5$ and $c = 1$, the relative losses of a false negative are equal to that of a false positive. If $r = 1$ then the Youden's index is equal to the Youden's index we used in the ordinal data section. The `coords()` function returns the coordinates of the ROC curve at one or several specified points and will calculate the closest top-left coordinates and the Youden criteria. The `ci.thresholds()` and `ci.coords()` functions can be used to find confidence intervals at specified coordinates.

```
# r1 is a ROC object

# return the coordinates of the ROC curve
# at specified point
pROC::coords(r1,
x = c(0.7,0.8),
input = "sensitivity")

pROC::coords(r1,
x = 0.6,
input = "specificity")

# All thresholds
pROC::coords(r1,
x = "all",
ret="sensitivity")

# find the best threshold - Youden method
pROC::coords(r1,
```

```
x="best",
best.method="youden")

# find the best threshold - closest top left
pROC::coords(r1,
x="best",
best.method="closest")

# specifying different weights.
pROC::coords(r1,
x="best",
best.method="youden",
best.weights=c(c,p))

# find best threshold and get CI for sens and spec
pROC::ci.thresholds(r1,
thres="best",
best.method="youden")

# obtain confidence interval for
# sensitivity at 90% specificity
pROC::ci.coords(r1,
x = 0.9,
input = "specificity",
ret ="sensitivity")
```

### 8.7.3   *Example*

We continue with the pulmonary nodule example from before. We
first refit the data and then find the best threshold according to the
Youden criteria.

```
data(IPNs, package  = "R4HCR")

r1 <- pROC::roc(cancer ~ rating,
direction="<", data = IPNs)
```

```
set.seed(1)
pROC::coords(r1,x="best",best.method="youden")

##   threshold specificity sensitivity
## 1      62.5   0.6888889   0.7727273

pROC::ci.thresholds(r1,thres="best",best.method="youden")

## 95% CI (2000 stratified bootstrap replicates):
##  thresholds sp.low sp.median sp.high se.low se.median se.high
##        62.5 0.5997    0.6889  0.7889 0.6818    0.7727  0.8636
```

According to the Youden criteria, the best threshold is 62.5, at which the sensitivity and specificity of the AI algorithm are 77.2% and 68.8%, respectively. Confidence intervals for sensitivity and specificity are 68.2–86.4% and 60.0–78.9%. We do not use the estimates of the median sensitivity and specificity. The random number seed is set because the confidence intervals are calculated using a bootstrap routine. The previous analysis was based on a prevalence of $p = 0.5$ and an equal cost of $c = 1$. We can change prevalence and cost parameters using the **best.weights** argument.

```
set.seed(11)
## equal costs (c=1), but prevalence p = 20%
pROC::coords(r1,x="best",best.method="youden",
best.weights=c(1,0.2))

##   threshold specificity sensitivity
## 1      86.5   0.9666667       0.375

## with c= 10
pROC::coords(r1,x="best",best.method="youden",
best.weights=c(10,0.5))

##   threshold specificity sensitivity
## 1      22.5   0.11111           1
```

Changing the prevalence parameter to 0.2, from the default of 0.5, increases the weight $r$ to 4, and has the effect of selecting a higher, more specific threshold (86.5 vs. 62.5). In our second example, we set the prevalence back to the default 0.5 and instead set $c = 10$. Now,

$r = 0.1$ and this has the effect of selecting a lower, more sensitive threshold of 22.5.

## 8.8 Problems and exercises

(1) A test for sepsis in bursitis was conducted in 17 patients with septic bursitis and 19 with non-septic bursitis. The test was positive in all 17 septic bursitis patients and negative in 17 of 19 non-septic bursitis patients (Stell and Gransden, 1998).

    (a) What kind of design is this study? What bias could this study be susceptible to, and how might it skew the results?

    (b) Calculate the sensitivity and specificity of the test, with a Wilson score confidence interval.

    (c) Derive the positive likelihood ratio for this test.

(2) The National SARS-CoV-2 Serology Assay Evaluation Group (2020) in the United Kingdom investigated the performance of five high-throughput commercial SARS-CoV-2 antibody immunoassays. The Oxford immunoassay detected 10 positives in 976 known negative samples and 531 positives in 536 laboratory-confirmed SARS-CoV-2 infection samples.

    (a) Calculate the sensitivity and specificity and exact 95% confidence intervals.

    (b) Suppose the true population prevalence of SARS-CoV-2 is 0.2%; what would be the positive predicted value of the Oxford immunoassay?

    (c) Interpret the meaning of the value obtained above.

(3) The following example is from Zhou *et al.* (2002). The results are gap measurements (the gap between valve strut legs) in patients who underwent elective surgery for heart valve replacement. Ten patients have fractured heart valve and ten patients have heart valve intact. It was hoped that gap measurements obtained by digital imaging could help identify fractured heart valves prior to surgery.

```
frac <- c(0.58,0.41,0.18,0.15,0.15,
0.1,0.07,0.07,0.05,0.03)
intact <- c(0.13,0.13,0.07,0.05,
0.03,0.03,0.03,0.0,0.0,0.0)
```

(a) Draw a vertical stripchart showing the distribution of gap measurements by heart valve status. Jitter the points to enhance the plot.
(b) Estimate the sensitivity and specificity at a threshold of 0.06.
(c) Draw an ROC plot of the heart valve data. Annotate the plot with point(s) that represent the sensitivity and specificity at the threshold(s) at which Youden's index is maximised.
(d) Estimate the AUC and 95% confidence interval. Is there enough evidence to suggest that gap measurements are better than chance?

(4) A study was conducted to assess the accuracy of an artificial intelligence (AI) algorithm for detecting pneumothoraces (PTXs) and its impact on the reporting performance of clinician groups routinely involved in the diagnosis and management of this condition. The study enrolled 18 readers, and each examined 393 images (205 without PTX and 188 with PTX) with and without the assistance of the AI. Each reader was required to rank each image using an eight-item confidence scale. The confidence scale represents the confidence (from lowest to highest) in the presence of a pneumothorax.

```
# Frequencies of confidence scores from
  lowest to highest. .
present <- c(176,312,185,54,64,246,539,1808)
absent <- c(1416,1617,461,40,24,43,53,36)
```

Using R,

(a) compute the sensitivity and false positive rate for each possible decision threshold,
(b) estimate and plot the smooth and empirical ROC curve for these data,

(c) calculate the area under the curve (AUC) and 95% confidence interval.

(5) This question is adapted from Zhou *et al.* (2002). Magnetic resonance angiography (MRA) is a non-invasive test to detect cerebral aneurysms. Of asymptomatic patients with a family history of aneurysms, 20% are thought to have an undetected aneurysm, whereas the figure is thought to be 0.02% in the general population. Suppose the test (MRA) has a positive likelihood ratio of 4. What is the positive predictive value for a person with a family history and a positive predictive value for the general population?

(6) Diagnosing acute appendicitis in children is challenging. A range of diagnostic tools is available to the clinician, including signs and symptoms such as rebound tenderness and nausea, clinical risk scores, and blood tests. Imaging options include abdominal and appendix ultrasonography. This question uses data that originate from a cohort study of children and adolescents aged 0–18 years admitted with abdominal pain and suspected appendicitis to a tertiary children's hospital in Germany over three years. For this question, treat the diagnosis variable `DiagnosisByCriteria` as the reference standard and delete missing observations case-wise. The data can be downloaded from https://github.com/i6092467/pediatric-appendicitis-ml/blob/main/app_data_clean.Rda, and the source paper is by Marcinkevics *et al.* (2021).

(a) Calculate the sensitivity and specificity (with 95% confidence intervals) of rebound tenderness for diagnosing appendicitis.

(b) Investigate whether 'migratory pain' might be useful in ruling in or ruling out appendicitis. Use appropriate diagnostic accuracy metrics to back your argument.

(c) Test whether there is a difference in specificities between lower abdominal pain (right) and migratory pain; is there any evidence to support that they are not equal?

(d) The variable `WBCinUrine` is an ordinal score with levels `none`, `+`, `++`, and `+++`. Tabulate this variable with the outcome (DiagnosisByCriteria) and assess its potential to discriminate cases of appendicitis with controls (people without appendicitis). Confirm your findings by calculating the sensitivity and specificity for each possible threshold.

(e) White blood cell count is predictive of appendicitis in some studies. Using an ROC approach, find the threshold that maximises Youden's index. Report the sensitivity and specificity of WBC for appendicitis at this threshold. Repeat the calculation, but this time weight the cost of a false negative to be twice that of a false positive.

(f) `AlvaradoScore` and `PediatricAppendicitisScore` are examples of clinical scores for appendicitis in children. Use these data to perform ROC analysis on the two scores, and test whether there is a difference in diagnostic performance.

(g) Is there any evidence to suggest that the two appendicitis scores are different if the focus is on the regions of the ROC curve that correspond to thresholds with low rates of false positives (e.g., no more than 30%). Find a suitable test to evaluate this hypothesis.

# Supplementary material

The supplementary material includes solutions to problems and exercises.

Online access is automatically assigned if you purchase the ebook online via www.worldscientific.com. If you have purchased the print copy of this book or the ebook via other sales channels, please follow the instructions below to download the files:

1. Register for an account or log in at: www.worldscientific.com/.
2. Go to: https://www.worldscientific.com/r/q0506-supp or scan the QR code below.

3. Download the files from: https://www.worldscientific.com/ worldscibooks/10.1142/q0506#t=suppl.

For subsequent access, simply log in with the same login details in order to access.

For enquiries, please email: sales@wspc.com.sg.

# Bibliography

Agresti, A. (1996). *An Introduction to Categorical Data Analysis*, 1st edn., Wiley, Hoboken, NJ.

Agresti, A. (2007). *An Introduction to Categorical Data Analysis*, 2nd edn., Wiley, Hoboken, NJ.

Agresti, A. and Min, Y. (2002). Unconditional small-sample confidence intervals for the odds ratio, *Biostatistics* **3**(3), pp. 379–386.

Altman, D. G. (1990). *Practical Statistics for Medical Research*, Chapman & Hall/CRC, Boca Raton, FL.

Altman, D. G. (1998). Confidence intervals for the number needed to treat, *British Medical Journal* **317**(7168), pp. 1309–1312.

Bååth, R. (2012). The state of naming conventions in R, http://journal.r-project.org/archive/2012-2/RJournal_2012-2_Baaaath.pdf.

Barnett, V. (1981). *Elements of Sampling Theory*, Hodder and Stoughton, London.

Bhattacharyya, G. K., Johnson, R. A. and Neave, H. R. (1970). Percentage points of some non-parametric tests for independence and empirical power comparisons, *Journal of the American Statistical Association* **65**(330), pp. 976–983, http://www.jstor.org/stable/2284602.

Bland, M. (1995). *An Introduction to Medical Statistics*, 2nd edn., Oxford Medical Publications, Oxford.

Bland, J. M. and Altman, D. G. (1996a). Measurement error proportional to the mean, *British Medical Journal (Clinical Research Edition)* **313**(7049), pp. 106–106, https://doi:10.1136/bmj.313.7049.106.

Bland, J. M. and Altman, D. G. (1996b). Statistics notes: Measurement error, *British Medical Journal* **312**(7047), p. 1654, https://doi:10.1136/bmj.312.7047.1654.

Bland, J. M. and Altman, D. G. (1996c). Statistics notes: Measurement error and correlation coefficients, *British Medical Journal* **313**(7048), p. 41, https://doi:10.1136/bmj.313.7048.41, http://www.bmj.com/content/313/7048/41.abstract.

Bland, J. M. and Altman, D. G. (1999). Measuring agreement in method comparison studies, *Statistical Methods in Medical Research* **8**(2), pp. 135–160, https://doi:10.1177/096228029900800204.

Braun, W. J. and Murdoch, D. J. (2007). *A First Course in Statistical Programming with R*, 1st edn., Cambridge University Press, Cambridge, UK.

Bustamante-Marin, X. M. and Ostrowski, L. E. (2017). Cilia and mucociliary clearance, *Cold Spring Harbor Perspectives in Biology* **9**(4), https://doi:10.1101/cshperspect.a028241.

Carobene, A., Guerra, E., Locatelli, M., *et al.* (2018). Biological variation estimates for prostate specific antigen from the European biological variation study; Consequences for diagnosis and monitoring of prostate cancer, *Clinica Chimica Acta* **486**, pp. 185–191, https://doi.org/10.1016/j.cca.2018.07.043.

Carstensen, B., Simpson, J. and Gurrin, L. C. (2008). Statistical models for assessing agreement in method comparison studies with replicate measurements, *The International Journal of Biostatistics* **4**(1), https://doi.org/10.2202/1557-4679.1107.

Chapelle, N., Martel, M., Barkun, A. N., *et al.* (2022). Relative risk rather than absolute risk reduction should be preferred to sensitise the public to preventive actions, *Gut* **71**(6), pp. 1045–1046, https://doi:10.1136/gutjnl-2021-324689, https://gut.bmj.com/content/71/6/1045.

Croswell, J. M., Kramer, B. S., Kreimer, A. R., *et al.* (2009). Cumulative incidence of false-positive results in repeated, multimodal cancer screening, *Annals of Family Medicine* **7**(3), pp. 212–222, https://doi:10.1370/afm.942.

Doll, R. and Hill, A. B. (1964). Mortality in relation to smoking: Ten years' observations of British doctors, *British Medical Journal* **1**(5396), pp. 1460–1467 concl, https://doi:10.1136/bmj.1.5396.1460.

Dyer, C. (2025). Professor Roy Meadow struck off. *BMJ*. **331**(7510):177, https://doi:10.1136/bmj.331.7510.177.

Efron, B. and Tibshirani, R. (1994). *An Introduction to the Bootstrap*, Chapman & Hall/CRC, Boca Raton, FL.

Everitt, B. (2006). *Medical Statistics from A to Z*, 2nd edn., Cambridge University Press, Cambridge UK.

Everitt, B. S. (2021). *Medical Statistics from A to Z: A Guide for Clinicians and Medical Students*, Cambridge University Press, Cambridge, UK.

Fraser, C. G. (2013). *Biological Variation: From Principles to Practice*, AACC Press, Washington DC.

Gallagher, J. (2006). The F test for comparing two normal variances: Correct and incorrect calculation of the two-sided p-value? *Teaching Statistics* **28**(2), pp. 58–60, https://doi.org/10.1111/j.1467-9639.2006.00244.x.

Gelman, A. and Hill, J. (2007). *Data Analysis Using Regression and Multilevel/Hierarchical Models*, repr. with corr., 3. print. edn., Analytical Methods for Social Research, University Press, Cambridge UK.

Glas, A. S., Lijmer, J. G., Prins, M. H., *et al.* (2003). The diagnostic odds ratio: A single indicator of test performance, *Journal of Clinical Epidemiology* **56**(11), pp. 1129–1135, https://doi:10.1016/s0895-4356(03)00177-x.

Goss, P. E., Ingle, J. N., Alés-Martínez, J. E., *et al.* (2011). Exemestane for breast-cancer prevention in postmenopausal women, *New England Journal of Medicine* **364**(25), pp. 2381–2391.

Gøtzsche, P. C. and Jørgensen, K. J. (2013). Screening for breast cancer with mammography, *Cochrane Database of Systematic Reviews* **2013**(6), p. Cd001877, https://doi:10.1002/14651858.CD001877.pub5.

Greenland, R. K. J. S. and Lash, T. L. (2008). *Modern Epidemiology*, 3rd edn., Wolters Kluwer Health/Lippincott Williams & Wilkins, Philadelphia, PA.

Holland, W. W., Bailey, R. and Bland, J. M. (1978). Long-term consequences of respiratory disease in infancy, *Journal of Epidemiology & Community Health*, **32**(4), pp. 256–259.

Hollander, M., Chicken, E. and Wolfe, D. A. (2014). *Nonparametric Statistical Methods*, Wiley Series in Probability and Statistics, John Wiley & Sons, Inc., Hoboken, NJ.

Howick, J., Zhao, L., McKaig, B., *et al.* (2022). Do medical schools teach medical humanities? Review of curricula in the United States, Canada and the United Kingdom, *Journal of Evaluation in Clinical Practice* **28**(1), pp. 86–92, https://doi.org/10.1111/jep.13589.

Hutton, J. (2000). Number needed to treat: Properties and problems, *Journal of the Royal Statistical Society: Series A (Statistics in Society)* **163**(3), pp. 381–402.

Jones, N., Oke, J., Marsh, S., *et al.* (2023). Face masks while exercising trial (merit): A cross-over randomised controlled study, *British Medical Journal Open* **13**(1), p. e063014, https://doi:10.1136/bmjopen-2022-063014.

Julious, S. A. and Mullee, M. A. (1994). Confounding and Simpson's paradox, *British Medical Journal* **309**(6967), pp. 1480–1481.

Khan, H., Khawaja, M. R., Waheed, A., *et al.* (2006). Knowledge and attitudes about health research amongst a group of Pakistani medical students, *BMC Medical Education* **6**, pp. 1–7.

Kim, R. Y., Oke, J. L., Pickup, L. C., *et al.* (2022). Artificial intelligence tool for assessment of indeterminate pulmonary nodules detected with CT, *Radiology* **304**(3), pp. 683–691, https://doi.org/10.1148/radiol.212182.

Kirkwood, B. and Sterne, J. (2010). *Essential Medical Statistics*, 2nd edn., Essentials Ser., John Wiley & Sons, Incorporated, Hoboken, NJ.

Labrecque, J. A., Hunink, M. M., Ikram, M. A., *et al.* (2021). Do case-control studies always estimate odds ratios? *American Journal of Epidemiology* **190**(2), pp. 318–321.

Lennox, B. R., Palmer-Cooper, E. C., Pollak, T., *et al.* (2017). Prevalence and clinical characteristics of serum neuronal cell surface antibodies in first-episode psychosis: A case-control study, *Lancet Psychiatry* **4**(1), pp. 42–48, https://doi:10.1016/s2215-0366(16)30375-3.

Li, M., Gao, Q. and Yu, T. (2023). Kappa statistic considerations in evaluating inter-rater reliability between two raters: Which, when and context matters, *BioMed Central Cancer* **23**(1), p. 799, https://doi.org/10.1186/s12885-023-11325-z.

Liljequist, D., Elfving, B., and Roaldsen, K. S. (2019) Intraclass correlation — A discussion and demonstration of basic features. *PLoS ONE* **14**(7): e0219854, https://doi.org/10.1371/journal.pone.0219854.

Low, P. M., Luk, C. K., Dulfano, M. J. and Finch, P. J. (1984). Ciliary beat frequency of human respiratory tract by different sampling techniques, *American Review of Respiratory Disease* **130**(3), pp. 497–498, https://doi: 10.1164/arrd.1984.130.3.497.

Mai, P. L., Khincha, P. P., Loud, J. T., *et al.* (2017). Prevalence of cancer at baseline screening in the National Cancer Institute Li-Fraumeni syndrome cohort, *The Journal of the American Medical Association Oncology* **3**(12), pp. 1640–1645.

Marcinkevics, R., Reis Wolfertstetter, P., Wellmann, S., Knorr, C. and Vogt, J. E. (2021). Using machine learning to predict the diagnosis, management and severity of pediatric appendicitis, *Frontiers in Pediatrics* **9**, p. 662183.

McGill, R., Tukey, J. W. and Larsen, W. A. (1978). Variations of box plots, *The American Statistician* **32**(1), pp. 12–16, http://www.jstor.org/stable/268 3468.

McGraw, K. O. and Wong, S. P. (1996). Forming inferences about some intraclass correlation coefficients. *Psychological Methods* **1**(1), p. 30.

Miller, D. K. and Homan, S. M. (1994). Determining transition probabilities: confusion and suggestions, *Medical Decision Making* **14**(1), pp. 52–58, https://doi:10.1177/0272989x9401400107.

Montgomery, D. C. (2001). *Introduction to Statistical Quality Control*, 6th edn., John Wiley & Sons Inc., New York, Chichester.

Mood, A. M., Graybill, F. A. and Boes, D. C. (1974). *Introduction to the Theory of Statistics*, 3rd edn., McGraw-Hill International Book Company, Tokyo, Japan.

Moroney, M. J. (1953). *Facts from Figures*, 2nd edn., Penguin Books, Harmondsworth, Middlesex, England.

Murrell, P. (2011). *R Graphics*, The R Series, CRC Press, Boca Raton, FL, London, New York.

Müller, R. and Büttner, P. (1994). A critical discussion of intraclass correlation coefficients, *Statistics in Medicine* **13**(23–24), pp. 2465–2476.

Noordzij, M., van Diepen, M., Caskey, F. C., *et al.* (2017). Relative risk versus absolute risk: One cannot be interpreted without the other, *Nephrology Dialysis Transplantation* **32**(2), pp. ii13–ii18, https://doi.org/10.1093/ndt/gfw465.

Pawitan, Y. (2001). *In All Likelihood*, Statistical Modelling and Inference Using Likelihood, Clarendon Press, Oxford.

Perkins, N. J. and Schisterman, E. F. (2006). The inconsistency of 'optimal' cutpoints obtained using two criteria based on the receiver operating characteristic curve, *American Journal of Epidemiol* **163**(7), pp. 670–675, https://doi:10.1093/aje/kwj063.

Rosen, L. (2013). An intuitive approach to understanding the attributable fraction of disease due to a risk factor: The case of smoking, *International Journal of Environmental Research and Public Health* **10**(7), pp. 2932–2943.

Sattar, N. and Preiss, D. (2017). Reverse causality in cardiovascular epidemiological research: More common than imagined? *Circulation* **135**(24),
pp. 2369–2372.

Schrag, D., Beer, T. M., McDonnell, C. H., *et al.* (2023). Blood-based tests for
multicancer early detection (pathfinder): A prospective cohort study, *Lancet*
**402**(10409), pp. 1251–1260, https://doi:10.1016/s0140-6736(23)01700-2.

Senn, S. (2005). Dichotomania: An obsessive compulsive disorder that is badly
affecting the quality of analysis of pharmaceutical trials, *Proceedings of the
International Statistical Institute*, 55th Session, Sydney.

Shen, S.-W., Reaven, G. M. and Farquhar, J. W. (1970). Comparison of
impedance to insulin-mediated glucose uptake in normal subjects and in
subjects with latent diabetes, *The Journal of Clinical Investigation* **49**(12),
pp. 2151–2160, https://doi:10.1172/JCI106433.

Shepherd, J., Blauw, G. J., Murphy, M. B., *et al.* (2002). Pravastatin in elderly
individuals at risk of vascular disease (prosper): A randomised controlled
trial, *Lancet* **360**(9346), pp. 1623–1630.

Shrout, P. E. and Fleiss, J. L. (1979). Intraclass correlations: Uses in assessing rater reliability, *Psychol Bull* **86**(2), pp. 420–428, https://doi.10.1037//
0033-2909.86.2.420.

Siegel, S. (1956). *Nonparametric Statistics for the Behavioural Sciences*, McGraw-
Hill Series in Psychology, McGraw-Hill Kogakusha, Tokyo, Japan.

Sim, J. and Wright, C. C. (2005). The kappa statistic in reliability studies:
Use, interpretation, and sample size requirements, *Physical Therapy* **85**(3),
pp. 257–268, https://doi.org/10.1093/ptj/85.3.257.

Skrabanek, P. and McCormick, J. S. (1990). *Follies and Fallacies in Medicine*.
The Tarragon Press, Glasgow.

Spiegelhalter, D., Abrams, K. and Myles, J. (2004). *Bayesian Approaches to Clinical Trials and Health-Care Evaluation*, Wiley, Hoboken, NJ.

Stell, I. M. and Gransden, W.R., 1998. Simple tests for septic bursitis: compara-
tive study. *BMJ*, **316**(7148), pp.1877–1880.

Thisted, R. A. (1988). *Elements of Statistical Computing*, Chapman & Hall, New
York.

Thomas, E. J. and Cooke, I. D. (1987). Impact of gestrinone on the course of
asymptomatic endometriosis. *British Medical Journal (Clinical Research
Edition)* **294**(6567), pp. 272–274.

Tufte, E. R. (2001). *The Visual Display of Quantitative Information*, 2nd edn.,
Graphics Press, Chesire, CT.

Tukey, J. W. (1977). *Exploratory Data Analysis*, Behavioral Science: Quantitative
Methods, Addison-Wesley Publishing Company, Reading, MA.

van Smeden, M. (2022). A very short list of common pitfalls in research design,
data analysis, and reporting, *Peer-Reviewed Reports in Medical Education
Research* **6**, p. 26, https://doi:10.22454/PRiMER.2022.511416.

Venables, W. and Ripley, B. D. (2000). *S Programming*, 1st edn., Statistics and
Computing, Springer, New York.

Venables, W. N. and Ripley, B. D. (2002). *Modern Applied Statistics with S-PLUS*,
4th edn., Springer Science & Business Media, New York.

Venkatraman, E. S. and Begg, C. B. (1996). A distribution-free procedure for comparing receiver operating characteristic curves from a paired experiment, *Biometrika* **83**(4), pp. 835–848.

Vogel, V. G., Costantino, J. P., Wickerham, D. L., *et al.* (2006). Effects of tamoxifen vs raloxifene on the risk of developing invasive breast cancer and other disease outcomes the NSABP Study of Tamoxifen and Raloxifene (STAR) P-2 trial, *JAMA* **295**(23), pp. 2727–2741, https://doi.org/10.1001/jama.29 5.23.joc60074.

Welch, H. G., Schwartz, L. M. and Woloshin, S. (2000). Are increasing 5-year survival rates evidence of success against cancer? *JAMA* **283**(22), pp. 2975–2978, https://doi:10.1001/jama.283.22.2975, https://www.ncbi.nlm. nih.gov/pubmed/10865276.

Zhou, X.-H., Obuchowski, N. A. and McClish, D. K. (2002). *Statistical Methods in Diagnostic Medicine*, Wiley Series in Probability and Statistics, Wiley-Interscience, New York.

# Index

www.ingramcontent.com/pod-product-compliance
Lightning Source LLC
Chambersburg PA
CBHW051304220526
45468CB00004B/1201